ALSO BY ANAHAD O'CONNOR

Never Shower in a Thunderstorm

ALWAYS
FOLLOW THE
ELEPHANTS

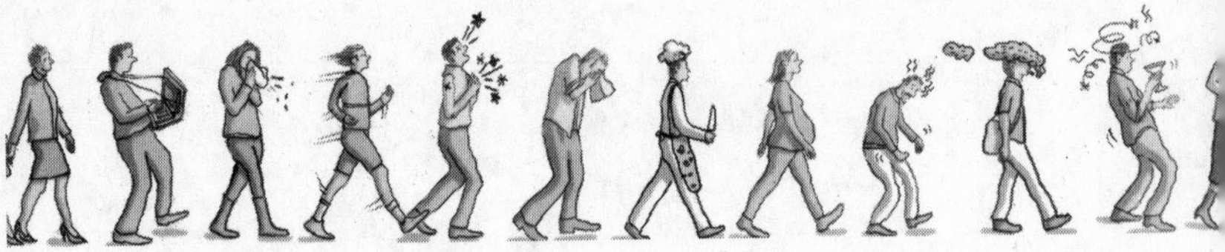

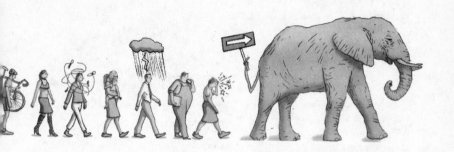

ALWAYS
FOLLOW THE
ELEPHANTS

*More Surprising Facts
and Misleading Myths
About Our Health and
the World We Live In*

ANAHAD O'CONNOR

TIMES BOOKS
Henry Holt and Company
New York

Times Books
Henry Holt and Company, LLC
Publishers since 1866
175 Fifth Avenue
New York, New York 10010
www.henryholt.com

Library of Congress Cataloging-in-Publication Data

O'Connor, Anahad.
    Always follow the elephants : more surprising facts and misleading myths
about our health and the world we live in / Anahad O'Connor.—1st ed.
        p. cm.
    Includes bibliographical references and index.
    ISBN-13: 978-0-8050-9000-0
  1. Medicine, Popular.   2. Health—Miscellanea.   I. Title.

    RC82.O26 2009
    613—dc22   2009005216

Henry Holt books are available for special promotions and premiums.
For details contact: Director, Special Markets.
First Edition 2009
Designed by Meryl Sussman Levavi
Illustrations by Leif Parsons
Printed in the United States of America
10 9 8 7 6 5 4 3 2 1

To Steve, who came to me as a Big Brother, and guided me through life as a father. Thanks for all these years of loving friendship and guidance.

CONTENTS

INTRODUCTION

Like an old relationship that just had to end but was too good to stay away for long, once again it's on!

Almost two years ago, my unconventional quest at the *New York Times* seemed all but complete. I had spent three years tracking down and examining a panoply of medical quandaries, myths, and old wives' tales in my Tuesday column, "Really?" for the Gray Lady's science section. After publishing a book covering more than a hundred of the most popular and intriguing subjects—going so far as to dig up the bizarre origins of many of the established claims that guide our day-to-day lives—I was just about ready to kick up my feet, certain that I had left no stone unturned.

But no sooner had I completed that thought than I discovered that my reporter's shovel had plunged only so far into the ground of revelation. Still wet behind the ears after all these years. In countless e-mail messages from readers, I found myself showered with even more questions about medical bromides, health folklore, and homespun remedies. My job had only just begun.

Like a dentist stepping into his office on the morning after Halloween, I knew I had my work cut out for me. Turns out the most surprising part about hunting down and holding up all sorts of rumors and urban legends to the light of scientific scrutiny is discovering just how many there really are out there.

As I quickly realized, some I had missed because they were thrown into circulation by recent events, like the questions about the 2004 tsunami that callers to NPR and other radio stations were anxious for me to answer. How it is that virtually no elephants and other animals perished in that disaster—is it true they all sensed it coming and got away early? Other questions had been around for years but simply never crossed my desk, or my mind, for that matter. Why on Earth is it so unbelievably hard to swat a fly? Still others had been bouncing around in my head for some time, but I never pursued them because, ahem, I write for a family paper and had good reason (until now) to skirt some more embarrassing subjects—like: Can sex be substituted for a workout? And do Kegel exercises really work?

Then there were those that I, like most people, had always accepted (perhaps too naively) as fact. Should you really tilt your head back to stop a nosebleed? And are hot drinks really any good for a cold or the flu?

As we saw in *Never Shower in a Thunderstorm*, some of these claims and conventional wisdoms carry weight and others are just plain nonsense. But which ones? It took countless hours of digging through medical journals and databases, and what seemed like an infinite amount of time pulling the experts away from their labs and Bunsen burners, all so I could nail down the best, scientifically endorsed answers to these pesky curiosities. What follows are the straight, in-depth, unbiased, and unadulterated facts. Not to mention some absurd fun and an abundance of trivial (and not so trivial) knowledge that could make you the star of any cocktail party. And by the way, as you'll soon find out, there really is a reason why you should always follow the elephants. . . .

ALWAYS
FOLLOW THE
ELEPHANTS

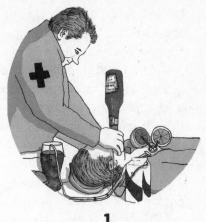

1
KITCHEN FIRST AID
Do-It-Yourself Doctoring

This is a chapter I was born to write.

My childhood was so jam-packed with spills and nasty injuries—enough for a special double episode of *America's Funniest Home Videos*. I stumbled through burns, bruises, broken bones, bloody noses, bike crashes, and bizarre animal attacks—not to mention the occasional high-speed baseball to the side of the head, sans helmet, of course. To this day I sometimes discover faded scars whose provenance are untraceable, and I have yet to meet a barber who doesn't comment on the unusual number of quarter-inch, gash-shaped bald spots peppered over the back of my head.

All of which means I spent an inordinate amount of time in my mother's medicine cabinet, sifting through bottles of rubbing alcohol and hydrogen peroxide, Neosporin and Bacitracin, in search of something to soothe the countless injuries inflicted on me by this harsh world. I may not have been the only child who kept baseball cards in one pocket of his Velcro wallet and Band-Aids and sterilizing wipes in the other. But I was probably the only one who considers that to have been field research.

Now I find myself wondering how many of those first-aid techniques and medicines were really worth their salt. Think about it for a moment: basic first aid is one of the few areas of medicine that has remained virtually the same for the past eighty years. The essential components of any first-aid kit—sterile dressings, wipes, a tube of ointment, bandages, cold packs, hydrocortisone, and a pain reliever—haven't changed since Charles Lindbergh was named *Time* magazine's debut "Man of the Year."

Of course, some might argue that this is not necessarily a bad sign. More than a few medical techniques that were introduced ages ago have stood the test of time. In the past few decades, for example, a growing number of doctors have employed flesh-eating maggots and bloodsucking leeches in high-tech surgeries—practices that were long thought of not only as outdated relics of a bygone era but, let's face it, disgusting. But leeches, it seems, are expert at removing excess blood from surgically reattached appendages. And maggots can clean up wounds better than almost anything else known to man, serving as unsightly little parasitic vacuum cleaners. These two practices, among other previously discarded medical techniques, are so widely used in operating rooms that in 2005 the U.S. Food and Drug Administration began discussions on how to regulate them, just like any other medical device.

But conversely, a number of first-aid methods that have been around for ages have turned out to be tried but not so true. In my years as a health reporter, I've uncovered evidence that the old way of treating a snakebite—suck out the poison, spit it out, and grab a tourniquet—can cause further damage (better to rush to a clinic to get antivenin); that treating a bee sting by scraping out the stinger is wrong (better to yank it out as quickly as possible, since time is all that matters); and that letting a cut or scrape "breathe" and get some air can do more harm than good (it creates a dry environment that promotes cell death).

So with that in mind, and my vast collection of scars and old wounds guiding me, I put some of my favorite first-aid tips and techniques to the test. Here are the results.

CAN A GLASS OF WARM MILK CURE INSOMNIA?

Like a soothing old blanket or the cool side of a favorite pillow, a glass of warm milk is thought to have the magical ability to carry you off to dreamland with a smile (and perhaps a milk mustache) on your face. It's a belief that dates back more than a thousand years. Jewish scholars appear to have been the first on record positing a relationship between milk and the onset of sleep. The Talmud, the collection of Jewish laws and traditions that dates as far back as A.D. 200, notes that "after eating fish, cress, and milk," you should "occupy your body and not your bed," lest you hit the sheets and fall into a deep sleep.

Centuries later, those who embraced the notion that milk leads to sleepiness pointed out that milk is chock-full of tryptophan, the sleep-inducing amino acid that is also well-known for its presence in another food thought to have sedative effects: turkey.

But whether milk has any special ability to induce sleep is debatable, and studies suggest that if it does, the role of tryptophan may be only a small part of it.

To have any soporific effect, tryptophan has to break the blood-brain barrier—a major hurdle when the tryptophan is consumed as part of a meal. In the presence of other amino acids and nutrients, tryptophan ends up fighting—largely unsuccessfully—to make its way across the blood-brain barrier. The more amino acids a meal contains, the harder it is for tryptophan to complete its journey to the brain.

Two things have to happen for tryptophan to have an effect: it must be consumed either by itself and on an empty stomach or in the presence of mostly carbohydrates, which stimulate the pancreas to release insulin. A surge of insulin, in turn, causes other amino acids to leave the bloodstream, freeing up room for tryptophan and allowing it more opportunities to reach the brain and be converted into serotonin, the chemical that ultimately sedates you.

A study by researchers at the Massachusetts Institute of Technology demonstrated this effect in 2003. When a group of subjects fasted overnight and then had a protein-rich food in the morning—like milk—the scientists found that the tryptophan in their bloodstreams was less likely to reach the brain. The trick, the study found, was to add some carbohydrates—say, by adding a little sugar to the milk—which caused the subjects' insulin levels to climb, ultimately allowing more tryptophan to be converted into serotonin.

But don't expect that to be the final word. National surveys by sleep researchers have shown that many people swear by plain old milk as a sleep aid and are reluctant to give it up. And they may in fact be seeing an effect—the placebo effect, that is. That's because anything that causes relaxation can lead to drowsiness, whether it's the soothing embrace of that fuzzy old blanket or the thought that the milk in your stomach will soon lull you to slumber.

Psychology can also have the opposite consequence. Lying in bed and brooding about your insomnia can keep you just as awake and alert as a shot of hot espresso. Instead, read a dull book, write a letter, or listen to some soft music—anything to take your mind off your frustrations and allow your brain's sleep centers to kick in.

CAN EATING GINGER CURE MOTION SICKNESS?

Whether on a ship, in a car, or on an airplane, most people have experienced the miseries of motion sickness. While the cause is always the same—conflicting sensory signals going to the brain—the list of potential remedies is vast.

One of the oldest is ginger, a traditional Chinese herb that's been touted as a remedy for motion sickness for decades. Major airlines started serving ginger ale on flights shortly after their inception for that very reason, and many airlines still make a habit of having it available during flights.

It may be hard to imagine any airline doing much of anything right when it comes to food. But on this front, at least, they were right. Using a spoonful of ginger as a miracle cure for motion sickness is backed by ample evidence: several studies have found it to be highly effective.

One study in the journal *Lancet* illustrated the medicinal qualities of ginger in an unusual and amusing way. The scientists recruited thirty-six people who were highly susceptible to motion sickness and on separate occasions had them ingest three different things: capsules of powdered ginger on one day, Dramamine (an antinausea medication) on another, and a placebo on yet another. Then, twenty minutes later, they were put in chairs and spun in circles for as long as six minutes.

Picture scientists in white lab coats throwing a group of queasy, skeptical subjects into chairs, then taking turns spinning them around and around—smiles and laughter filling the room, I'm sure. It sounds more like playtime in grade school than good science, but it was all in the name of medical research. And the scientists reached a solid conclusion: taking ginger delayed the onset of sickness about twice as long as taking the medication. The scientists also found that half the subjects who took ginger lasted the full six minutes, compared with none of those given the placebo or the medication.

Another study by Danish scientists echoed those findings, albeit through more traditional means. It looked at eighty naval cadets prone to seasickness and found that those given 1 gram of ginger powder suffered less nausea in a four-hour period than those given a placebo.

Precisely how ginger works is unclear, but it may have something to do with one of its active compounds, 6-gingerol, which is known to aid digestion and settle upset stomachs. Whatever the mechanism, it may be a good idea to pack some ginger on your next boat trip.

SHOULD YOU TILT YOUR HEAD BACK TO TREAT A NOSEBLEED?

Most of us know the correct way to stop a nosebleed: Lean your head back, use your thumb and index finger to clasp your nose, and apply pressure until the bleeding stops.

But what most people know about treating nosebleeds is wrong. Tilting the head back, a technique widely considered proper first aid, can actually create complications by allowing blood into the esophagus. It risks choking, and it can cause blood to travel to the stomach, possibly leading to severe stomach problems.

"Not only will the swallowed blood conceal the actual degree of bleeding but it will also act as an irritant to the stomach, causing haematemesis and occasionally malaena," warn the authors of a study that appeared in the *Journal of Accident and Emergency Medicine*. Haematemesis is a fancy medical term for vomiting blood, and malaena refers to the passage of black, tarry stool. A simple nosebleed, at least in my estimation, would be preferable to either of these.

That should be reason enough to follow the *proper* procedure. The American Academy of Family Physicians says the best treatment is to sit down, lean forward, and keep your head above your heart, which lessens the bleeding. Leaning forward also helps drain the blood from the nose and keeps it out of the esophagus. Use a bowl to catch blood, if necessary.

You can also stop the bleeding by using your thumb and index finger to squeeze the soft tissue just below the bridge of your nose for five to ten minutes. A cold compress or ice pack placed across the bridge of the nose can also help. If all of this fails and the bleeding lasts for more than twenty minutes, or the nosebleed was caused by a blow to the head, it could be more serious, in which case you should seek medical attention.

Over the years, readers have written to the *Times* to float some of their own ideas for treating nosebleeds. Pierre Clavel of Ithaca passed along the following technique: "A family friend once stopped my nose from bleeding by rolling a small piece of tissue and sticking it behind my upper lip. It worked almost immediately, and has ever since. I now use this with my kids, and although it looks silly, it is very effective."

Then there was Moom Luu of New York City, who suffers from what can only be described as a most unusual allergy: "I had chronic nosebleeds for years, especially after drinking a cold soda. When I was thirteen, my stepfather, a physician, showed me the most effective way to stop a nosebleed: He took a small piece of gauze or half a cotton ball, soaked it with cool water, then wrung it out. Then he had me gently put it up the bleeding nostril for a few minutes. I've been doing it since 1986, whenever my nose decides to get back at me for having a soda."

I can't endorse either of those techniques, but if they work, I can't see how they might cause any side effects. I suppose I won't know until the next time I suffer an unfortunate blow to the nose and have a chance to find out.

CAN A PAT OF BUTTER SOOTHE A BURN?

It's soft, smooth, rubs on easily, and it's always nearby when you suffer a burn in the one room of the house where burns are most likely to occur, the kitchen. So it's no wonder why butter has long had advocates as a salve for minor burns.

But save the butter for your toast. Because butter and margarine retain heat and irritate wounds, they can prevent proper healing and make your injury a breeding ground for bacteria. The Centers for Disease Control and Prevention specifically warns against using butter because of the risk of causing infection, and it also advises steering clear of many other convenient burn "remedies," which run the gamut from egg whites to toothpaste.

A few home remedies seem like obviously bad ideas, such as rubbing jalapenos on a wound, dressing it with potato slices, or smearing it with mustard (Grey Poupon, I presume?). But at least one offbeat remedy, honey, has held up well.

In studies of quick and easy treatments to soothe mild burns, scientists have found that honey has antibacterial and anti-inflammatory properties that may promote healing. One study in 2006, examining results of more than a dozen previous studies, found that small, nonserious burns healed faster, on average, when treated with gauze and a dash of honey than those treated with antibiotic creams and other dressings. A separate report published earlier found similar results. Analyses of the compounds in honey suggest the healing properties have something to do with antimicrobial agents known as inhibines, which are abundant in the stuff.

Medical experts say the tried-and-true method for healing

small burns remains applying a wet compress, immersing the burn in cool water, and then covering the area with a sterile, non-adhesive bandage. But for those who prefer using natural remedies to soothe discomfort, honey appears to be a sweet option.

What about aloe vera gel?

Another skin-care remedy, aloe vera, has been used ever since the Greek physician Diosco advocated it to soothe and treat burns in the first century A.D. Even the Bible contains references to aloe vera, the "bitter herb," and the gel from this succulent plant was said to have been part of the secret to Cleopatra's transcendent beauty: the gel kept her skin looking smooth and younger than its true age. Many historians contend that her captivating appearance played no small role in her conquests of some of the world's most powerful men, from Julius Caesar to Mark Antony, as she rose to political dominance.

So synonymous is aloe vera with healthy skin that today it's added to everything from tissue to sunscreen and shampoo. But even though it's been around for millennia, it's only in recent years that scientists have trained the lenses of scientific scrutiny on aloe vera to determine whether it actually lives up to its reputation.

Some have found that aloe contains a small number of anti-inflammatory compounds, and may act as an antibacterial and antifungal agent. But studies that have looked at its effects on minor and moderate burns have largely produced conflicting findings.

In 2007, for example, a study in the journal *Burns* analyzed data from four controlled clinical trials involving a total of 371 patients, some of whom were treated with topical aloe vera and others with placebo. The authors found that patients in the aloe vera group appeared to have slightly shorter healing times—a difference of about eight days in some cases—but the evidence was not persuasive, and they recommended further research.

In another study, scientists examined aloe vera's effectiveness by applying it to second-degree burns and comparing it to other treatments. They found that the aloe vera "hindered the healing process" when compared to a common antibacterial cream. Then in 2008, another study that looked at aloe vera applied to burns over the course of six weeks found that it decreased "subdermal temperature within the skin," but did not reduce bacterial counts or speed the regeneration of skin.

The bottom line of all these studies: you're better off saving the aloe for rough skin instead of first-degree burns. If it worked for Cleopatra . . .

CAN URINE CURE A JELLYFISH STING?

Nothing can ruin a day at the beach quite like a jellyfish sting. The gelatinous creatures—technically not fish, but members of the phylum Cnidaria—sneak up with no warning, have the unpleasing consistency of a bowl of cold Jell-O, and more often than not leave their victims crouched in excruciating pain.

Jellyfish are known, as well, to strike rather frequently. But while such attacks are common, the methods for treating the stings vary widely—and many remedies may do far more harm than good. As much pain and distress as an attack can set off, the last thing you want to do is to aggravate your suffering. Who knows how many people over the years have twisted and contorted themselves—to get in the right, ahem, position—in the name of that old saw about urine relieving jellyfish stings. Or how many people have asked *others* to do the deed. If only they had known beforehand that urine is generally not acidic enough to make a difference—unless of course you factor in the possibility that the overwhelming shame and humiliation that follows might serve as a distraction from the pain.

In fact, many other well-known methods for relieving jellyfish stings—for instance, rubbing alcohol, ammonia, and meat tenderizer—don't work either. Even rinsing a sting with freshwater can be a bad idea, because the change in pH between salt water and freshwater can prompt the release of more venom.

But one exception is the application of vinegar, which, according to several studies, can deactivate the venomous nematocysts that jellyfish release. A study published in the *Medical Journal of Australia* showed that removing any tentacles left by a jellyfish, then dousing an injured body part with commercial vinegar or its crucial ingredient, acetic acid, could alleviate pain and "rapidly and completely" prevent the release of more venom. "Most other substances tested proved less effective, and some actually stimulated the firing of nematocysts," the authors wrote.

(One important note: you need to get medical attention if you are attacked by a Portuguese man-of-war, the jellyfish's more dangerous relative—which can be identified by its extremely long tentacles [stretching as long as thirty-three feet] and its large, bluish air sac, or sail [which resembles the sail of a man-of-war naval vessel]. That is especially true if your symptoms include muscle pain, shortness of breath, backache, and hives.)

After dousing the jellyfish nematocysts with the proper solution, it's important to remove them and scrape any small pieces away with a razor, a credit card, or another object with a flat edge. If the scraping isn't working too well, try smearing shaving cream over the injured area and then scraping once again. A study published in the journal *American Family Physician* in 2004 found this works well.

Of course, after simmering in vinegar and shaving cream, a shower might be in order. Best to hold off on washing with freshwater for at least thirty minutes after the attack. The smell may not be very pleasant, but it beats writhing in agony.

Does CPR require mouth-to-mouth?

There are some emergency techniques that are so common (and so commonly depicted in television shows) that even people who have never been trained in them know what they involve. The basic steps in cardiopulmonary resuscitation (CPR) fit that bill: everyone knows CPR involves delivering a series of chest compressions combined with mouth-to-mouth resuscitation.

The practice goes at least as far back as 1911, when it was outlined in the first edition of the *Boy Scout Handbook*. Some argue that it dates back even further, saying versions of the method were promoted by doctors in the 1800s, and that even the Bible contains a passage, in the book of Kings, in which Elisha, the Hebrew prophet, uses some version of CPR to resuscitate a Shunnamite child:

> And he went up, and lay upon the child, and put his mouth upon his mouth, and his eyes upon his eyes, and his hands upon his hands: and he stretched himself upon the child; and the flesh of the child waxed warm. Then he returned, and walked in the house to and fro; and went up, and stretched himself upon him: and the child opened his eyes.

It is hard to argue with a practice that dates back millennia. But virtually every medical technique evolves over time, and CPR may be no different. That's because in recent years, very good evidence has emerged suggesting that the mouth-to-mouth part of CPR may be unnecessary—and even harmful. That's because in most cases of cardiac arrest, the victim's body has enough oxygen to keep organs functioning for several minutes. Mouth-to-mouth simply delivers more oxygen, while chest compressions perform the more vital task of pumping blood to vital organs.

In one of the largest studies of traditional CPR versus compression-only CPR (also called cardiocerebral resuscitation, or CCR), researchers looked at more than four thousand cases of cardiac arrest and found that patients were more likely to recover without brain damage if their rescuers had focused on chest compressions alone. Published in the *Lancet* in 2007, the study found that 22 percent of people who received chest compressions alone survived with good neurological function, compared with 10 percent who received traditional CPR.

Those findings echoed those of a randomized study published in the *New England Journal of Medicine* in 2000, which compared what happened when emergency telephone dispatchers instructed bystanders at the scene of a cardiac arrest to administer either traditional CPR or compression-only CPR. Overall, 279 people were randomly instructed to administer the traditional technique and 241 were instructed to give only chest compressions. Not only did the patients who received chest compressions alone have slightly better survival rates, their rescuers had an easier time: it took the emergency dispatchers 1.4 minutes less to rattle off instructions than it took to relate instructions for traditional CPR.

When a person is unconscious and on the brink of dying, those eighty-four seconds can make the difference. Experts have also argued that bystanders are more likely to intervene and use CCR than CPR, perhaps because most of us tend to be just a *little* skittish about doing mouth-to-mouth on a complete stranger.

The evidence is such that in 2008, the American Heart Association took the bold step of endorsing compression-only CPR, saying in a statement, "Hands-only CPR is acceptable to perform on victims of sudden cardiac arrest. Compressions should be of high quality with minimal interruptions and can increase a victim's chance of survival."

I guess you might say, "To everything there is a season, a time for every purpose under the sun."

Can super glue heal wounds?

Call it the secret life of super glue.

During the Vietnam War, emergency medics began using the all-purpose glue to seal battle wounds in troops headed for surgery. The glue was so good at stemming bleeding that it was credited with saving many lives.

Nowadays, professional athletes often close small cuts with super glue or similar adhesives to get back in the game in a hurry. Veterinarians use it regularly on their furry patients. Backpackers and outdoorsmen are known to pack a tube of the stuff before heading out into the wilderness. And many people keep a tube around the house—in the medicine cabinet instead of the hardware drawer—to help them out of a medical pinch. It is believed that the glues—made from the chemical cyanoacrylate—not only stop bleeding quickly, but also lead to less scarring.

If you're one of the millions of people who have accidentally spilled some of the glue on your hand and spent days trying to remove it, then you have a good idea of what it can do to help wounds—namely, it acts as an adhesive barrier that prevents air, dirt, and other substances from getting in. And all the while it keeps the skin joined together before eventually flaking off.

Another advantage: it works in many places where regular bandages won't, like the tips of your fingers or on your knuckles.

So should you keep some super glue in your first-aid kit? Probably not. Studies have found that although such super adhesives can be useful in emergencies, they can also irritate the skin, kill cells, and cause other side effects, particularly when used on deep wounds.

There is a safer alternative. In 2001, the Food and Drug Administration approved a similar, antibacterial form of the substance called 2-octyl-cyanoacrylate, which is marketed as Dermabond. It has all the benefits of super adhesives but without the toxic effects, and many surgeons make frequent use of it in the operating room in place of sutures and staples for closing wounds.

Apparently it helps to avoid the "ouch" factor that comes from removing stitches. Now if only we could find another use for that old bottle of wood glue that's been sitting in your house for thirty years.

CAN CHEWING GUM PREVENT HEARTBURN?

Chomping wads of bubble gum is supposed to be the province of adolescents. I said good-bye to Bazooka Joe around the same time I gave up video games, Wiffle ball, and spin the bottle (well, maybe not that last one). But as a health reporter I often discover quirky cures for common ills, and bubble gum, which was perhaps bound to pop up, is one of the more unusual.

Take the list of home remedies for heartburn, a condition that afflicts as much as 7 percent of the world's population (amounting to more than 85 million people). Heartburn has long been the target of improvised treatments, many of them unproven. When and why chewing gum was first proposed as a cure for it is not clear, but something about it seems to stick: it has been on the list for decades. But is there any truth to it?

Heartburn, known more fondly among medical types as gastroesophageal reflux, occurs when fluids in the digestive tract reverse course and travel from the stomach to the esophagus. At first glance, it is not terribly easy to see how chewing gum could have any effect on this process. So when scientists set out to study whether a stick or two of spearmint could counter it, they assumed the answer would be no. Instead they found good evidence that saliva was the key: chewing stimulates fluids that neutralize wayward stomach acid and help force it back to the stomach.

In a study published in the *Journal of Dental Research* in 2005, for example, researchers had thirty-one people eat heartburn-inducing meals and then asked some of those subjects to chew sugar-free gum for thirty minutes. Acid levels after the meals were significantly lower when the participants chewed gum. A similar study in 2001 compared the effects of chewing gum after a large breakfast in people with gastroesophageal reflux and in those without it. It found that the beneficial effects of chewing gum on heartburn lasted up to three hours, "with a more profound effect in refluxers than in controls." Another option is antacid chewing gums, which have been found even more effective after a meal than chewable tablets.

While gum seems to have the most scientific backing of all the home remedies for heartburn, there are some other unconventional ones: plain and simple walking, for example, provides some help, though not as strong as that of chewing gum, and not as long-lived.

So heartburn sufferers of the world rejoice. Relief may be as simple as a quick trip to the candy store.

CAN YOU SWALLOW YOUR TONGUE DURING A SEIZURE?

One problem with old wives' tales and medical myths is that they can sometimes lead well-meaning people to do ill-advised things.

People who are prone to seizures may know this better than anyone. Armed with the adage that a person in the midst of a seizure can swallow his or her tongue, Good Samaritans will often try to help by forcing an object into the victim's mouth to keep the person from choking.

The notion of choking on your own tongue has been firmly cemented by depictions in movies and television, perhaps most viscerally in *The Silence of the Lambs*, when the serial killer Hannibal Lecter talks an inmate in the cell beside his into swallowing his tongue, resulting in the man's death. It's a frightening and persistent belief, but much like the story of Hannibal Lecter, a fictitious one.

In reality, swallowing your tongue is virtually impossible. In the human mouth, a small piece of tissue called the frenulum linguae, which sits behind the teeth and under the tongue, keeps the tongue firmly in place, even during a seizure.

One person who spends more time than he'd like to trying to dispel this myth is Ryan Brett, the director of education for the Epilepsy Institute of New York City. People who witness a seizure, he said, often reach for a wallet, a spoon, or a dirty object to stick in the person's mouth, much to the chagrin of epilepsy patients. As if enduring a seizure were not difficult enough, having filth jammed into your mouth is an added indignation.

Brett frequently conducts first-aid workshops designed to disabuse people of this myth, and says that people are often shocked to learn that the technique can do more harm than good. "The only thing that happens when something is put in the mouth is you end up cutting someone's gums or injuring the teeth," he said.

Instead, the best way to help a person during a seizure is to roll the person on one side to drain fluids from the mouth, cushion the head to prevent cranial injuries, and seek medical help if necessary. In the meantime, be sure that no one attempts to forcefully hold the person down, which can cause injuries like a broken collarbone. "When a person is convulsing and their muscles are moving involuntarily, you don't want to restrain them," Brett said.

Just give the person some room. Many times, the seizure will pass and the person will regain normal functioning.

DOES BREATHING INTO A PAPER BAG HELP YOU IF YOU'RE HYPERVENTILATING?

If there is one universal symbol for a quick and easy way to calm a person who is overexcited and hyperventilating, it has got to be the brown paper bag.

We've all seen the method—perhaps in a gym class, though definitely in a movie or two. A person is floored by some shocking news or unexpected event, starts breathing rapidly and heavily, and needs to sit down and hold a brown paper bag to his or her mouth to relax and catch a breath. It's a method known in the medical literature as "rebreathing"—or paper-bagging it, in the P.E. classes I come from—and it's been recommended as a way to ease hyperventilation. Some doctors even keep paper bags in their offices for that very reason. But most medical studies and experts argue that the method, though widely accepted as proper first aid, is dangerous and should be retired.

The idea behind the brown paper bag technique is to increase carbon dioxide levels in the bloodstream. Breathing too fast and too deeply, a hallmark of hyperventilation, causes the body to expel too much carbon dioxide, and "rebreathing" air that has been exhaled into a bag helps restore that lost carbon dioxide.

But the problem is that a number of medical conditions, like asthma and heart attacks, can be confused with hyperventilation, and in some cases what the person really needs is more oxygen. Increasing carbon dioxide when the person is gasping for oxygen can have deadly results. And as someone who suffered from asthma as a child and is no stranger to hyperventilating—and paper-bagging it—this realization nearly took my breath away.

Imagine my surprise when I found a study published in the *Annals of Emergency Medicine* that described three cases in which people accidentally died because of a brown paper bag. In each case, the victims thought they were hyperventilating but were actually having heart attacks, and they reached for paper bags thinking it would help them, when in fact they ended up losing more and more oxygen and ultimately making matters worse.

Another study published in the *Journal of Behavioral Medicine* took a different approach. The scientists compared what happened when they "provoked" a group of lucky subjects into hyperventilating, then had them breathe into a paper bag in some cases and breathe into what they described as a "semiclosed tube system" in other cases. The subjects weren't told that in at least one case the tube system was actually open.

Breathing into a bag, the results showed, was no better at easing hyperventilation than breathing into the open tube. So there really is no advantage to paper-bagging it. For best results, it's better to simply stay calm, take a seat, and practice breathing very slowly and deliberately. Counting can also help pace your breathing.

And make sure the only brown paper bag in sight is the one holding your lunch.

IS HYDROGEN PEROXIDE THE BEST TREATMENT FOR CUTS AND SCRAPES?

It is a staple in medicine cabinets everywhere, a first-line treatment for the small cuts and scrapes that a hazardous world can inflict upon our skin. But does hydrogen peroxide make a difference?

According to most studies of its effectiveness, not really. Parents and school nurses might insist otherwise, but researchers have found that hydrogen peroxide has little ability to reduce bacteria in wounds and can actually inflame healthy skin cells that surround a cut or a scrape, increasing the amount of time wounds take to heal.

In a study published in the *Journal of Family Practice* in 1987, scientists compared the effects of various topical treatments by taking a group of volunteers, administering several small blister wounds on each of their forearms, and then infecting their wounds with bacteria. After applying a different treatment to each wound, they measured bacterial amounts and rates of healing. They found that hydrogen peroxide did not inhibit bacterial growth and that wounds treated with the antibiotic bacitracin healed far more quickly.

Another study, in the *American Journal of Surgery*, looked at more than two hundred people who had appendectomies and found that hydrogen peroxide did not reduce the risk of infection at the site of their incisions. But according to the American Medical Association, hydrogen peroxide does have at least one benefit: it can help dislodge dirt, debris, and dead tissue in some wounds.

Instead of pouring the hydrogen peroxide, rinse small wounds with water and apply an antibiotic to promote healing.

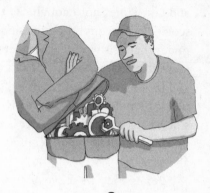

2
REGULAR
MAINTENANCE

Your Body, as Time Goes By

They say the only certainties in life are death and taxes. But I've got a few qualms with that statement.

For one thing, at least the grim reaper is kind enough to strike us only once, which is something that cannot be said about the IRS. And second, I am fairly sure about a few other certainties in life. One is that someone, at some point, will send you an e-mail message asking you to wire money to Nigeria. Another is that life is filled with a certain set of questions that invariably confront us at specific times in our lives, much like the various stages of life itself.

The one exception is infancy, because at that point, we are little more than miniature, pleasure-seeking ids. But as toddlers and adolescents we begin to ask inevitable questions. One of the first puzzled me for some time because I could not get a straight answer: exactly why are we are all given three names? Are first and last names not enough? As I eventually learned, after being scolded numerous times, the singular purpose of a child having a middle name is so parents can let them know when they are *really* in trouble. Soon I was struck by a series of questions that plague—and in some cases haunt—most children. Exactly what will happen if I swallow this massive piece of gum in my mouth? And is something wrong with me or is all that pain in my legs on some mornings nothing but the consequences of growth spurts, as Mom always said?

Before long we move on to our teenage years, a period dominated by obsessions that are superficial but nonetheless of some importance. Most of us, for the first time in our lives, are suddenly bombarded with constant stress—the stress of balancing the difficulties of high school, the vagaries of friendships, and the mental and sexual frustrations suddenly triggered by an avalanche of hormones. Like many teens, I wondered at times what all this stress was doing to me, and particularly to my skin, which seemed to have more eruptions than Old Faithful. Not exactly what you want when you're navigating the heavily social and superficial world of high school.

Then comes the early adult years, that time in life when you manage to stay in impeccable shape despite a diet that would kill a small horse, and a strategy for daily exercise that includes "cure hangover" as step number one. But it's all in good fun, because pretty soon after that you reach a stage in life where you start relying on your joints to tell you the weather, you leave any club you go to by 10 P.M. to beat "the rush," and you still make late night trips to the pharmacy—but for FiberCon, not birth control. Yes, that's right. It's in these middle decades that you start trying to recover from all of the damage you did as a reckless teen and twenty-year-old: Can drinking lots of water make my skin look healthier? Can vitamin E erase all those scars? And how on Earth can I kick this smoking habit?

As the years go by you enter your later years, the twilight of your life, a time when an afternoon of adventure involves a book, a cup of tea, and a rocking chair. And for a *really* crazy time, you break out the Scrabble. But it's at this time that you also find yourself asking another set of questions. Will a daily aspirin protect me from Alzheimer's? And what are some hidden signs and causes of a stroke?

With the cycle of life and its inevitable questions in mind, let's begin a revealing search for some answers . . .

IS IT DANGEROUS TO SWALLOW CHEWING GUM?

For generations, parents have told their children never to swallow chewing gum, lest it sit undigested for days, weeks, or even years in their digestive tracts.

The refrain has been around for—well, it turns out that no one can really say for sure. The first commercial chewing gum, called the State of Maine Pure Spruce Gum, was made and sold in 1848 by a man from Maine named John B. Curtis, after he noticed loggers chomping on spruce resin. But he was only capitalizing on a habit that had been around for centuries, practiced by various cultures on various continents. The ancient Greeks chewed resin from the mastic tree, which they called *mastiche*, and the ancient Aztecs and Mayans chomped on an extract from evergreen trees that they called *chicle*, which later gave Chiclets, the famous brand of pocket gum, its name.

Regardless of its source, what is universal about gum—other than its popularity among humans—is that it ordinarily does not pose as much of a hazard to your gut as it does to your hardwood floors. Like a marble making its way through a plumbing pipe, swallowed chewing gum typically passes through the digestive tract without harm and is eliminated at the same rate as other foods.

But complications can and do occur. The medical literature contains a number of case reports describing people, mostly small children, who developed intestinal obstructions because they had a habit of swallowing their gum, one piece after another, taken down straight like shots of Bubblicious, which collected and congealed, forming huge, immovable masses.

A 1998 study in the journal *Pediatrics*, for example, described three children who came to a clinic with intestinal pain, constipation, and other symptoms, and were found to have small masses of chewing gum in their guts. One was a four-year-old boy who "always swallowed his gum after chewing five to seven pieces each day." His parents, unfortunately, had been using chewing gum to reward him for successful potty training.

Another was a four-year-old girl who had a habit of swallowing her gum just to get her parents to give her more. Clever, perhaps, but the results were none too pretty. Her experience at her pediatrician's office marked what may have been the first time that a doctor had ever removed anything from a patient's body that produced what was described in the report as "a taffy-like trail." I'll leave the rest of the case report to your imagination. (For those who want the clinical details, consult the notes at the end of the book.)

Three other studies, including one in the *American Journal of Diseases of Children*, describe similar cases. In most, the young patients were fine after removal of the rainbow-colored obstructions. While the phenomenon is rare, these studies should serve as cautionary tales for parents of small children, particularly when those children have a strong fondness for gum.

In other words, all children.

ARE GROWING PAINS CAUSED BY GROWTH SPURTS?

There's something disconcerting about watching a child sitting around, apparently feeling fine, suddenly clutch an arm or leg and wince in pain as if hit by an invisible projectile. These inexplicable aches and pains can strike in the middle of the day or late at night for no obvious reason. For decades, doctors have dismissed them as the normal, harmless signs of growing in small children, giving them the innocent-sounding nickname "growing pains," which is the medical profession's way of saying "fuhgettaboutit."

As many as 50 percent of all children experience these mysterious pains at some point in their lives, mostly in the muscles of the arms and the legs. Usually the diagnosis of growing pains is one of exclusion: when doctors cannot find any other cause or explanation for the pains, they use this catchall term. Most textbooks simply attribute the pains to the stretching of leg muscles, caused by the rapid growth of bones—and leave it at that. Despite widespread acceptance of this explanation, there is virtually no evidence that it's true.

Recent studies have found instead that the pains result from brittle bones and physical activity, in particular overuse from running, climbing, and jumping during the day. And there is something that can be done to stop them. In 2005, a team of scientists decided to figure out whether there was something in particular about the bones of children with growing pains that predisposed them to the phenomenon, so they recruited thirty-nine children with symptoms and compared them with a control group. After ultrasound tests, the researchers found that the children in the pain group had significantly decreased "bone speed of sound"—a measure of bone strength and breakability—indicating that these children had relatively weak bones. The scientists concluded that the kids were suffering from a "local overuse syndrome." In other words, children are generally very active—running, jumping around, roughhousing, for example—and in those with weaker bones, this can lead to muscle pains and soreness. A number of studies have had similar results.

If you're an adult, imagine getting knocked around on the jungle gym, jumping rope, chasing friends around a playground for hours on end, or playing an intense game of baseball one day. Wouldn't you expect some aches and pains over the next couple of days?

The analogy is not perfect, but the gist is that we often expect kids to get banged up, take a few whacks here and there, and shake it off. In adults, we call the pain that strikes in the ensuing days delayed-onset muscle soreness. In children, we shrug it off as growing pains. In this age of spiraling rates of childhood diabetes and obesity, children need to be encouraged to get as much exercise as possible, but it's also worth being aware of injuries caused by overuse.

Rather than dismiss the pains, parents can alert their pediatricians or try massages and a pain reliever.

One study also found that children with growing pains were more likely to have a parent with a history of restless legs syndrome, suggesting that in some cases, there may be an underlying condition that's been overlooked.

CAN TOO MUCH STRESS CAUSE ACNE?

Chronically bad skin or the occasional nasty breakout can be a major source of stress. That much is known. But what about the reverse?

Although scientists have suspected for some time that emotional stress can cause or worsen acne, the evidence for a causal relationship has mostly been weak, stemming instead largely from anecdotal observations. I've known people over the years who've said that their acne flares so terribly during stressful times that a blind person could read their face. If stress causes acne, and acne causes stress, then that is setting many people up for one vicious cycle.

What we know for sure is that acne is largely influenced by genetics and hormonal fluctuations, which is why it often strikes during puberty, pregnancy, and menopause, when our hormones jump up and down like a five-year-old throwing a tantrum. The medical field had long been divided on whether stress plays any role, with many scientists saying there was no connection what-soever. However, multiple studies in recent years have confirmed the link, and the largest on the subject to date was able not only to illustrate the relationship, but also to provide an explanation.

The study, by researchers at Wake Forest University in North Carolina, followed ninety-four high school students with mild or moderate acne for several months. Acne is generally associated with high levels of sebum, the oily substance that coats the skin and protects the hair. Because sebum levels are known to wax and wane with variations in weather, the scientists decided to conduct the study in a place where the temperature and humidity rarely change: Singapore.

Using a standard measure of stress, the researchers showed that in periods of high emotional strain—like before major exams—the students were 23 percent more likely to experience breakouts. At the same time, their sebum production did not vary much whether they were experiencing high or low stress, in-dicating that levels of that substance had little or no role. Instead, the results may have more to do with inflammation. Other studies have shown that stress can provoke inflammation—and at its root, acne, of course, is an inflammatory disease. There is also some evidence that psychological stress slows the healing of wounds, which can prolong the amount of time it takes your skin to recover from a breakout.

So forget about chemical peels and facials. For good skin, try back massages and stress balls.

CAN VITAMIN E ERASE A SCAR?

Home remedies for scar removal run the gamut from lemon juice to the wondrous aloe vera. But one that stands above the rest—in popularity at least—is vitamin E.

Depending on whom you ask, a little vitamin E dabbed on the skin can make all sorts of blemishes vanish like props in a magic act. It supposedly removes stretch marks, clears away scars, and even heals wounds. Discovered in 1922, it can be found widely now in all sorts of moisturizers and creams.

But according to most studies, its scar-busting properties are overstated. One of the largest studies to investigate the claim was published in 1986 in the *Journal of Burn Care and Rehabilitation*. In it, scientists followed a group of 159 people who had suffered burns over the course of a year, randomly selecting some to regularly apply vitamin E to their scars and others to use a different topical cream. Those in the vitamin E group showed no noticeable improvement in the size, thickness, or appearance of their scars by the end of the study.

In a 1999 study, scientists at the University of Miami followed a group of patients who had recently had minor surgery. Each patient was given two ointments labeled A and B—one with vitamin E, the other without—and told to apply each to a separate half of their scars twice daily for four weeks. After that, the scars were evaluated by the patients, the scientists, and an independent observer. The vitamin E not only had no beneficial effect on the appearance of the scars, it made matters worse. Almost a third of the patients had an allergic reaction known as contact dermatitis, leading the authors to give vitamin E the thumbs-down.

Your best bet? After suffering a cut or small wound, avoid vitamin E and antibiotic ointments (which can also lead to swelling and contact dermatitis) and reach instead for plain old petroleum jelly. Apply it twice daily. And when that irksome scab has reared its hideous head, don't leave it be for too long. Most dermatologists recommend leaving a scab alone just long enough for the bleeding to stop. If left on much longer, you'll get a larger scar. You can remove it easily by soaking and then gently scraping it away. Just be sure to slather on some petroleum jelly afterward.

IS DRINKING LOTS OF WATER GOOD FOR YOUR SKIN?

By now, the old saw about drinking eight glasses of water a day has been thoroughly debunked. Much of the water we need comes in the form of food and various liquids, like tea, milk, and juice, so there's no need to squeeze a minimum of eight glasses of water into your day if you're already consuming other fluids and eating properly.

But a similar adage about needing lots of water for healthy skin persists.

Where or how the claim originated is not well known, though it may have something to do with the common notion that our bodies are 60 to 70 percent water, and therefore require plenty of water to keep our skin from drying out. Whether that's the basis is anyone's guess. It is clear, however, that there's also no real evidence that drinking anything more than recommended amounts of water is particularly beneficial to skin.

One study in 2007 on the effects of water consumption on healthy skin did show that drinking 500 milliliters of water, or roughly 2 cups, increased blood flow to the skin. A good sign, but there was no evidence that over time that could reduce wrinkles or improve complexion. Other studies have hinted that vitamin C might help prevent wrinkles, or that estrogen use in post-menopausal women might reduce dry skin and slow skin aging. But the evidence for each is limited, and estrogen therapy can have some side effects.

Dr. Margaret E. Parsons, an American Academy of Dermatology spokeswoman and a professor at the University of California at Davis, told me that while excess quantities of water will not specifically make your skin more supple or give it extra sheen, "if dehydrated, fine wrinkles certainly seem to show up a bit more."

"Staying appropriately hydrated is good for our general health and if we are eating and drinking what we should, our bodies are healthier and therefore our skin as well."

Her advice?

Always wear sunscreen, avoid cigarettes, and try to eat well. If your diet's not in good shape, there's a chance your skin won't be either.

CAN SMOKING ACCELERATE AGING?

A story I heard a while back nicely illustrates the relationship between smoking and aging.

Years ago, the tale goes, a reporter from New York traveled to a small town in the Midwest to write a breaking story. After filing the story and wrapping up for the day, the reporter stopped in a local diner for a meal, and chatted with a waitress who revealed that her town was home to the world's oldest man. Intrigued, and eager for another good story, the reporter quickly paid his tab and asked for directions to the man's home.

A short time later, when the reporter arrived, he found a frail, shriveled man in a straw hat, his lanky frame folded into a rocking chair on the porch. Gently, the old man swayed back and forth, with slow, turtle-like leisure.

After some light conversation, the reporter asked the man for his secret to health. "Every day," the man said, "I make sure to have a glass of whiskey followed by two packs of cigarettes."

"Wow! That's amazing," the reporter beamed. "Just amazing. Who would have thought, with everything we know, that this could be the Fountain of Youth!"

At this, the reporter leaned in closer. "So tell me sir," he said to the man, "exactly how old *are* you?"

"Just turned twenty-six," the man replied.

Okay, I concede that this tale contains more than a few questionable truths. But one grain of reality is that smoking does seem to accelerate the aging process, and by far the most striking reflection of this seems to be the impact it has on hair.

Epidemiological studies provide ample reason for dread. In the mid-1990s, a team of researchers looked at more than 600 men and women, half of them smokers, and found that, after controlling for age and other variables, a "significant" and "consistent" link between smoking and early graying. In 2007, another team studied the link in a group of 740 men between the ages of forty and ninety-one in Taiwan, a notable population because Asian men generally have low rates of hereditary baldness. After controlling for age and family histories, the researchers found a greater rate of hair loss among the smokers, a risk that grew with increasing smoking.

But hair loss is only one of the age-accelerating side effects. One fascinating study found that smoking has such a profound impact on wrinkles and other facial features that people who smoke for ten years or more can be identified by their facial appearances alone—a phenomenon that's been dubbed "smoker's face."

Then there are the rapid signs of aging that occur at the molecular level, the changes we can't see. Deep within our cells, the chromosomes that carry our genetic information are capped by repetitive strands of DNA called telomeres. These caps protect our sensitive chromosomes from damage, but as our cells age, our telomeres erode from wear and tear, like a pencil eraser that's been rubbed down to a nub. This leaves the chromosome in harm's way: shortened telomeres have been linked to chronic diseases like diabetes and atherosclerosis. And when enough telomeres in a cell disappear, the cell dies off. (When the cell doesn't die off, essentially going haywire, we call it cancer.)

Smoking, it turns out, accelerates the shrinking of telomeres and all the problems that go along with it. One study in the journal *Lancet* found that smoking a single pack of cigarettes in a year effectively caused the loss of about 18 percent of telomere length beyond what was normal. Interestingly, obesity also accelerated the loss of telomere length.

But on the particular issue of hair loss and premature graying, there remain some questions. One is whether the link is a result of tobacco toxins directly damaging the scalp, or perhaps the indirect result of severe smoking-related diseases that speed the aging process. Most scientists tend to support the notion that chemicals in smoke harm hair follicles and damage hormones. It remains to be seen from future studies precisely what the root (pun intended) cause is.

But either way, if an increased risk of chronic illness and disease—not to mention telomere shrinkage—are not reason enough for many smokers to consider quitting, then perhaps a message focused on hair instead of health may do the trick.

CAN ACUPUNCTURE HELP YOU STOP SMOKING?

Arturo Toscanini, the Italian musician, was one of the greatest conductors of all time. A man who was known for his exquisitely precise ear, his fierce musical intensity, and his photographic memory, he may very well have been not just the preeminent conductor of his time, but one of the greatest minds of the early twentieth century.

But on a more mundane level, Toscanini could be applauded for something else: in a turn-of-the-century culture in which smoking was not only accepted but encouraged, Toscanini was often asked how he managed to avoid picking up the habit despite its popularity among so many friends and colleagues. "I kissed my first girl and smoked my first cigarette on the same day," he was known to say. "I haven't had time for tobacco since."

If only the millions of people across the globe who pick up cigarettes for the first time every day could find similar distractions to help them shun the habit. Unfortunately, the strength of Toscanini's willpower is something else that many of us do not share and, to be fair, studies show that genetics strongly predisposes some people to be more susceptible to the effects of nicotine than others.

Which is why smoking cessation techniques have sprouted a multimillion-dollar industry. Nicotine patches, gum, and prescription medication are the usual avenues. But one of the more intriguing tools for smokers looking for a way to kick the habit is acupuncture. Smokers have been turning to the needle-based traditional Chinese medicine for decades, but does it actually work?

According to those who endorse it, acupuncture helps stimulate the release of endorphins and other brain chemicals, blotting out cravings and easing the symptoms of nicotine withdrawal. A 2006 survey by the Mayo Clinic found that about 27 percent of smokers looking to quit had tried acupuncture at least once, and many others said they hoped to try it in the future.

Most research, alas, suggests they could just as well try something else. One of the most extensive studies, published in the *Cochrane Database of Systematic Reviews*, looked at more than a dozen previous investigations, most comparing acupuncture with sham, or fake, acupuncture and other control conditions. The scientists who led the study found that acupuncture and similar interventions—acupressure and electrostimulation, for example—were better in the short term than no treatment at all, but that overall they were not very effective.

Still, other studies show that more than three-quarters of smokers will relapse a few times—no matter what. And because the effects of different techniques vary from one person to the next, most scientists recommend combining interventions, particularly using both those that involve behavioral modification and those that replace the nicotine source.

When you're looking to quit, among the most important first steps to take is setting a day or time to stop smoking completely. In the run-up to that moment, it helps to eliminate some craving-inducing cues, like the ashtrays and matches you keep in your car, on your desk, or on your side table. You can also prepare for the moment by gradually reducing the number of cigarettes you smoke in a day, and choosing cigarettes with less and less nicotine strength.

Keep in mind that in 2008 researchers at Harvard University found that it's easier to quit in groups. If a friend or colleague is looking to kick the habit, join forces: your odds of success will be higher.

And if that doesn't work, and you find that patches, gum, and medication are not quite doing the trick, consider taking a piece of advice that a friend once shared with me: "The best way to stop smoking is to carry wet matches."

Are lefties more prone to migraines?

As if left-handers did not have it hard enough.

Already burdened with the minor mishaps that arise from living in a world designed for the right-handed—lefties are known to have higher accident rates, particularly with power tools, scissors, and other gadgets (almost exclusively designed for right-handers)—

their lot in life seemed to worsen considerably in the 1980s. That was when an extensive study argued that southpaws had several times the risk of chronic headaches and immune disorders as their right-handed counterparts. The reason, it was theorized, had something to do with variations in fetal brain development, though no precise explanation was given.

The news left many southpaws scratching their heads, and in some cases running to the local pharmacy to stock up on ibuprofen. But it seems in the light of more evidence that all those right-handers who praised the findings were, in one sense at least, not right.

A raft of contradictory evidence suggests that the original study, though intriguing, was less fact than statistical artifact. In 2008, German scientists examined a group of one hundred patients who had received a diagnosis of migraine based on standards set by the International Headache Society. After finding no evidence of a link between handedness and migraines, the scientists pooled data from five other studies and conducted a meta-analysis. Still, there was no evidence of a relationship—a conclusion echoed by many similar studies.

Others have also looked into whether there is any relationship between left-handedness and increased risk of immune disorders, but produced largely inconclusive findings. Proponents argue that fetal exposure to high levels of testosterone could be responsible, and they point out that left-handedness is more common in men than in women, while critics say more research is needed.

If you happen to be one of the many southpaws who feel slighted, you've got a reason to perk up: you're in good company. While lefties make up less than 10 percent of the population worldwide, they claim more than a fair share of historical figures, creative geniuses, and recent American presidents:

Julius Caesar   Benjamin Franklin
Napoleon   Michelangelo

Lewis Carroll	James A. Garfield
Pablo Picasso	Herbert Hoover
Robert Redford	Harry S. Truman
Paul Simon	John F. Kennedy Jr.
Robert De Niro	Gerald Ford
Oprah Winfrey	Ronald Reagan
Ty Cobb	George H. W. Bush
Sandy Koufax	Bill Clinton
Martina Navratilova	Barack Obama

Of course, this list isn't scientific—think of all the average left-handers who *aren't* included.

CAN CRACKING YOUR NECK CAUSE A STROKE?

Cracking your neck is ideally supposed to relieve pain and tension, not cause it. But many years ago, neurologists began to notice a strange pattern among some of their younger stroke patients: they were suffering their strokes shortly after having been to chiropractors for neck-adjustment procedures.

Pretty soon, there seemed to be a good explanation. There are four major arteries that run through the neck: two carotid arteries in the front, and two vertebral arteries that run through the back. The vertebral arteries are particularly susceptible to injury, and a chiropractic technique called cervical spinal manipulation, which involves forcefully twisting the neck, is capable of providing the force necessary to tear or rupture those arteries. Since they feed blood directly to the brain, any damage to these arteries can set off a blockage or loss of blood that results in a stroke.

Strokes in people under the age of forty-five are fairly rare, and these cervical arterial dissections are a leading cause of them.

With a plausible biological explanation for this pattern in place, a number of studies soon followed, and their findings present a grim picture. One of those studies, conducted by scientists at Stanford University, surveyed 177 neurologists in California—a state with one of the highest rates of chiropractic procedures in the country—and revealed that the neurologists had treated fifty-five patients who suffered strokes shortly after seeing chiropractors. Another, published in the journal *Neurologist* in 2008, found that young stroke patients were five times more likely to have undergone neck-adjustment procedures within a week of their strokes than a control group. The study estimated an incidence of 1.3 cases of stroke for every 100,000 people under the age of forty-five who visit chiropractors for neck procedures. That may not sound like very many, but when you consider the millions of people who undergo chiropractic procedures every year, the numbers quickly add up.

Still, a number of other researchers have cast strong doubt on the link. Critics say that it's not a causal relationship, but a temporal one—in other words, a mere coincidence. How is that possible? A 2008 study in Canada provided a good illustration. It examined 818 cases of stroke linked to arterial dissections at the back of the neck that were treated at hospitals in Western Ontario over a nine-year period. Before their strokes, the younger patients who saw chiropractors were more likely to have complained beforehand of head and neck pain—two symptoms that commonly precede a stroke. That suggests that some of these patients may have suffered ruptures in their vertebral arteries without knowing it, and then when they experienced some of the symptoms, went to chiropractors looking for relief, thinking they simply needed a good neck adjustment. In the days or hours that followed, however, the rupture resulted in a stroke. And there's your coincidence.

So how might these younger patients have suffered these strange arterial dissections? The list of things that can cause them is surprisingly long and diverse. All it takes is a good twist or abrupt jerk of the neck, and in some cases simply keeping your neck in a hyperextended position for a prolonged period of time will do the trick. Causes include, but are not limited to, lifting heavy objects, practicing yoga, being in a car accident, undergoing medical procedures that require you to hold your neck way back (that includes dental procedures), and coughing, sneezing, and vomiting. Sports injuries are another common cause.

But the most bizarre? Getting your hair washed in a beauty salon, which requires you to keep your head held back for long periods of time. More than a half a dozen studies have reported cases of it, and doctors have dubbed it the beauty-parlor-stroke syndrome.

When it comes to cracking your neck and its relationship to strokes, neurologists say the risk is certainly real, but the extent of it is unclear. One way to lower the risk is to ensure that any chiropractor you visit is properly licensed, and to be alert for warning signs like severe headaches and neck pain. For people who enjoy the occasional neck-crack—or, for that matter, trip to the beauty salon—it's something to keep in mind.

CAN ASPIRIN LOWER YOUR RISK OF ALZHEIMER'S DISEASE?

Doctors have long said that an aspirin a day can help ward off heart attacks. In fact, older people at risk of cardiovascular problems are often told to pop a small amount of aspirin every day. But might that protection pertain not just to the heart, but also the brain?

There is good reason to think so. Aspirin is an anti-inflammatory medication, and Alzheimer's, put simply, is an inflammatory disease. When the disease—which affects about 10 percent of Americans—takes shape, enzymes in the brain cleave and tear apart certain proteins that, once broken down, morph into tangled masses of plaque known as amyloids. These plaques disrupt nerve signals and may even kill off nerves. Aspirin, and possibly other nonsteroidal anti-inflammatory drugs, or NSAIDs, may help slow or head off that process. Other NSAIDs include ibuprofen and naproxen. (Acetaminophen is not an anti-inflammatory agent.)

One vast analysis by researchers at the University of Toronto pooled the results of nine previous studies, involving about 15,000 people overall, and found that those who regularly took an NSAID lowered their risk of Alzheimer's by 30 percent. Another study in 2003 looked at 702 people—351 pairs of twins of the same sex—and found that those who took "high-dose aspirin had significantly lower prevalence of Alzheimer's dementia and better-maintained cognitive function than non-users." And still another study, which followed more than 3,000 seniors in Utah for almost a decade, found that those who started taking an NSAID on a regular basis in midlife had a reduced risk of cognitive decline after the age of sixty-five than their peers who didn't take the drugs.

There are plenty more studies in that category to cite. To be sure, as with any good debate in science, there are those on the opposite side who urge caution. They point to studies like one in 2007 by researchers at Brigham and Women's Hospital who followed more than six thousand women (aged sixty-five and older) for nearly a decade and concluded that taking 100 milligrams of aspirin every other day did "not provide overall benefits for cognition," when compared to a placebo. But that study had some qualifiers. The subjects were already older, and most proponents of aspirin intervention argue that it should be started in midlife, not later. Plus, the authors conceded that they found some benefits. The women assigned to take aspirin were "20 percent less likely to develop substantial decline in performance" on "category fluency," a test of language and mental abilities used to spot symptoms of dementia.

Because frequent use of aspirin can cause side effects like stomach bleeding and ulcers, doctors aren't quite ready to encourage every middle-aged person to start taking it to ward off Alzheimer's disease. But the evidence is such that anyone with a family history of Alzheimer's or dementia might want to consider small doses in midlife. That's especially the case when early symptoms seem to be cropping up. A big one is profound memory loss, which applies not just to misplacing keys and occasionally losing track of small details—heck, I'd forget my own pants some mornings if I didn't live on such a breezy street—but repeatedly missing important appointments, blanking on details about a conversation or a show you just watched, and forgetting meetings with close friends or relatives. Anyone who can start a sentence with "I've lost my way home so many times this year . . ." might be a good candidate.

When that's the case, it's time to see a doctor. And should you find yourself in that boat, may the following words of wisdom, a popular serenity prayer for seniors, bring you some consolation: "God grant me the senility to forget the people I never liked anyway, the good fortune to run into the ones I do, and the eyesight to tell the difference."

IS IT DANGEROUS TO BLOW YOUR NOSE WHEN YOU HAVE A COLD?

Blowing your nose to alleviate the oppressive feeling of stuffiness that you get with a cold is almost second nature. But some people argue it does no good, reversing the flow of mucus and packing it into the sinuses, which slows drainage rather than speeding it up.

To test the notion, Dr. J. Owen Hendley and other pediatric infectious disease researchers at the University of Virginia conducted computed tomography (CT) imaging scans and other measurements as people coughed, sneezed, and blew their noses. In some cases, the subjects were asked to expel an opaque dye that was dripped into their rear nasal cavities, which scientists could be sure had a uniform consistency—unlike those resistant mucus secretions.

Coughing and sneezing generated little if any pressure in the nasal cavities. But nose blowing generated enormous pressure—about seven to eight times the pressure produced by coughing or sneezing—and propelled mucus into the sinuses every time. Hendley said it was unclear whether this was harmful, but added that during sickness it could shoot viruses or bacteria into the sinuses—possibly causing further infection.

"Whether God intended us not to blow our noses, I don't know, but blowing your nose *will* propel mucus back into your sinus cavities," Hendley told me. "If I were a stronger person than I am, I would never blow my nose with a cold—but I'm not. The sniffing back, which my Momma told me is a bad idea, I do that when I can."

For all those nose-blowers out there, myself included, don't fret just yet. Blowing your nose is fine, so long as you do it the right way.

The proper method is to blow one nostril, said Dr. Anil Kumar Lalwani, chairman of the department of otolaryngology at the New York University Langone Medical Center. This prevents a buildup of excess pressure, which is a good rule for both nose-blowing and its involuntary cousin, the sneeze.

Is stifling a sneeze bad for you?

I still remember the first time I was told that holding in a sneeze could be harmful. I was ten years old, and a teacher who had just spotted me stifling a sneeze warned that I shouldn't make a habit of it. "You could burst a blood vessel," she warned me. To a ten-year-old with an outsize imagination, that conjured images of my head bursting like a supernova. In fear, I vowed from then on that I'd let my mighty nasal storms blow and stick to deflecting what I could with my hands.

In the years that followed, I heard that warning repeated over and over, but by various people citing various reasons—lung damage, neck injuries, eye problems, you name it. But while holding in a sneeze isn't exactly a great idea, the reasons to avoid it aren't so far-flung.

Think of it this way: sneezing is essentially our first line of defense against infection. It expels germs, bacteria, dust, pollen, and other irritants from the body. And this involuntary action succeeds in its mission with lightning efficiency. Some scientists place the speed of a typical sneeze at about ninety-five miles an hour, while others put it at nearly the speed of sound (sound travels at 767 miles an hour).

That's a lot of power!

So much power that holding in a sneeze would be a bad idea. The built-up pressure could in fact burst a blood vessel or cause damage to your ears and sinuses. And of course, you keep your body from doing exactly what it intended: remove germs and particles. Why go through all that trouble, and expose yourself to that much risk, when the alternative is so simple: just let it out!

Besides, there are other bodily functions you can repress, or at least attempt to, without the potentially dire consequences . . .

What about holding in a fart?

Strange as it may be, the disposition of flatulence isn't solely a modern concern. Some of history's greatest minds have given it their attention.

Hippocrates, the father of medicine, once exclaimed that "passing gas is necessary to well-being." And the Roman emperor Claudius, who reigned from A.D. 41 to 54, once passed a law allowing all Roman citizens "to pass gas whenever necessary," reportedly out of concern for the public health. The law was later reversed, until it fell out of favor.

While people have debated the dangers of holding in "ill wind" for millennia, modern biology suggests doing so does not pose a hazard; in fact, it might even be good for you. A study in 2008 found that hydrogen sulfide, the compound that's primarily responsible for the rotten-egg-like stench, helps lower blood pressure by relaxing blood vessels. The substance is naturally produced in the lining of blood vessels, but scientists are now looking for ways to incorporate it into new drug therapies for hypertension.

Unfortunately, if you're looking to knock a few points off your blood pressure by holding in your backfire, don't count on it. No matter how hard you try, it'll always come out eventually, whether at night, at inopportune moments, or simply when you attempt to relax. Even if you hold one in and it goes away, it won't stay away for long. The gas has simply traveled upward to the intestine and disappeared—temporarily. Because of peristalsis—the process by which the intestine contracts and squeezes its contents outward—it will return. And it has just as good odds of occurring in the form of an embarrassing one-gun salute.

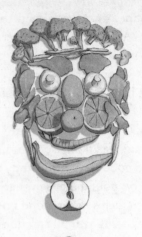

3
CALORIES COUNT

The Battle of the Bulge

Every day we fight a constant struggle, one that's carried out on two battlefields: the gym and the kitchen.

Of course, you've heard all the warnings about diet and exercise. You've heard the warnings against yo-yo dieting, yet listened eagerly to news about miracle menu plans hoping to find some morsel of willpower. You've had your fill of all the articles rattling on about the rising obesity epidemic, and you're all but exhausted of reading about the dangers of a sedentary lifestyle. You might even think you've become knowledgeable enough in these subjects to qualify as a registered dietitian. Good. But what's often lost in discussions of diet and exercise are answers to the seemingly mundane questions about the foods most of us still consume daily—from caffeine to butter to soft drinks and sugar—

and the ways in which most of us choose to fight the many calories those foods stack on our frames.

Investigating regular old food and workouts may at first appear so commonplace that it is at best a fleeting curiosity. But our relationship to food and exercise is far more intimate and extensive than many of us realize—especially in the case of food.

Food begins to exert an influence over us long before most people realize. It starts in the womb, when the food our mothers choose to send our way—across the placental bridge that connects us—affects our development. I am always amazed by studies showing, for example, that children born to mothers who drank lots of carrot juice while pregnant are likely to report carrots as a favorite food later on in life. Or that mothers who devour chocolate while pregnant give birth to children who become lifelong chocoholics. Consider, too, that pregnant women who step up their intake of fish, with its brain-building compounds like DHA, have children who generally score higher on motor and cognitive tests as toddlers than their peers who were born to non-fish-consuming mothers.

Your mom was eating for two when she carried you. What she ate, you did. And chances are it has had an effect on you that lasts to this day. Which probably explains my previously mysterious penchant for pickle and mustard sandwiches.

After we leave the cauldron of creation and make our debut, we continue to be shaped for life by the sustenance that flows through our bodies. Omega-3s in breast milk raise our IQ scores, while the foods that are slowly worked into our infant diets, from cow's milk to peanuts, influence the allergies we go on to develop. As we age, our diets continue to play subtle but significant roles in our development, our moods, our behavior, and our health.

It's the quirkier, everyday questions about foods, their calories, and their impact that intrigue me the most. It's the ones that confront us when we step into the kitchen, reach for our morning coffee, go out for a bite to eat, gather around a table for dinner, or perhaps even gear up for a jog. Does drinking tea reduce stress? Do sugary soft drinks *really* ramp up your energy or just make you crash? Can spicy meals ruin your sleep? What about your metabolism: can spicy foods rev it up? Is white meat healthier than dark?

And when all the eating is said and done, and we're looking to shed some much regretted calories, will we burn them off more efficiently on a soft and bouncy treadmill, or outside on the cold hard ground as nature intended? I don't know about you, but I'm suddenly feeling very curious . . .

IS WHITE MEAT HEALTHIER THAN DARK MEAT?

Every year, as millions of people gather around their dinner tables and prepare to carve up their Thanksgiving turkeys, an age-old question comes into play: set some pillows on the couch so you'll have a place to topple once your fork hits the table, or plan on fighting the food coma as you stumble half-consciously toward a bed? I always go with the couch, the closer option, as I've been known to give up on walking shortly after a massive meal.

But another question, one of slightly more import, also confronts the Thanksgiving feaster: dark meat or white?

Health experts have long advocated choosing white meat over dark, saying it contains less fat and fewer calories. So let's take a look at how the nutritional differences compare.

In general, what makes one cut of turkey—or any other type of poultry—darker than another is the type of muscle it contains. Meat is darker if it contains higher levels of myoglobin, a compound that enables muscles to transport oxygen, which is needed to fuel activity. Since turkeys and chickens are flightless and walk a lot, their leg meat is dark. Their wing and breast meat, conversely, are white.

Many people choose white meat over dark because of its lower caloric content. But according to the Department of Agriculture, an ounce of boneless, skinless turkey breast contains about 46 calories and 1 gram of fat compared with roughly 50 calories and 2 grams of fat for an ounce of boneless, skinless thigh. As you can see, the caloric differences are not so great, but dark meat has *double* the overall fat content of its white meat counterparts. Roughly two-thirds of the overall fat content of dark meat consists of polyunsaturated and monounsaturated fats (the good kinds), but the rest is saturated. (It's worth noting that this extra fat is the reason many people consider dark meat to be better-tasting.)

Still, dark meat has its benefits. Compared with white meat, it contains more iron, zinc, riboflavin, thiamine, and vitamins B_6 and B_{12}. Plus, both have less fat than most cuts of red meat, so you can't go wrong either way.

IS BROWN SUGAR HEALTHIER THAN WHITE SUGAR?

We all know that whole wheat bread is better for you than its bleached counterpart, and brown rice comes out on top over white—but can we say the same for brown and white sugars?

For as long as I can remember, brown sugar has been touted as the healthier, all-natural option for sugar lovers. Get the sweet flavor without the guilt—or at least not as much of it—the thinking went. But for the most part, you can chalk that up to clever marketing and plain and simple illusion. In reality, brown sugar—the type that beckons to you from diner countertops and supermarket shelves—is usually little different than white granulated sugar. Normally, molasses is separated and removed when sugar is created from sugarcane plants. Brown sugar is that ordinary table sugar, turned brown through the reintroduction of molasses.

In some cases, brown sugar—particularly when it is referred to as "raw sugar"—is sugar that has not been fully refined. But more often than not, manufacturers prefer to reintroduce molasses to fine white sugar, creating a mixture with about 5 percent to 10 percent molasses. They prefer this because it allows them to better control the color and size of the crystals in the final product. It's about aesthetics, not flavor, and certainly not health.

When it comes down to it, the two varieties of sugar are nutritionally similar. According to the Department of Agriculture, brown sugar contains about 17 calories per teaspoon compared with 16 calories per teaspoon for white sugar.

Because of its molasses content, brown sugar does contain certain minerals, most notably calcium, potassium, iron, and magnesium, which white sugar does not have. But since these minerals are present in only minuscule amounts, there's no real health benefit to using brown sugar. The real differences between the two are the effects they have on baked goods. Brown sugar tends to produce moister cakes, cookies, and muffins, while white sugar leads to crispier, lighter products.

A little baker's secret I picked up: try substituting dark brown sugar for white sugar in recipes that call for a lot of chocolate. The brown sugar produces a fudgier flavor. That's not a matter of health, but it sure tastes good.

IS MARGARINE HEALTHIER THAN BUTTER?

The debate has been around nearly since the invention of margarine—differences in flavor aside, is butter or margarine least likely to leave you with the aftertaste of guilt?

The confusion over the value of choosing butter or margarine persists for good reason. Butter, which has been used for millennia and dates at least as far back as 8000 B.C. in Mesopotamia, is made from animal products, making it high in the cholesterol and saturated fats that we know are strongly tied to heart disease. One landmark study of eighty thousand people in the *New England Journal of Medicine* found that every 5 percent increase of energy intake from saturated fat in a daily diet—compared to an equivalent energy intake from carbohydrates—was associated with a 17 percent increase in the risk of coronary artery disease.

Margarines, on the other hand, are usually made from a mixture of two types of oil: polyunsaturated vegetable oils like corn and canola oil, which contain very little in saturated fats, and tropical and fully hardened oils, which contain higher levels. Ultimately a typical brand of margarine will consist of no more than 50 percent saturated fat. Most people assume that makes margarine less of a hazard to your heart than butter.

But it's not that smooth. The process of turning polyunsaturated oils into semisolid table spreads creates trans fats, which are widely considered far worse than their saturated cousins. These are the artery-hardening fats that cities like New York and Philadelphia as well as the entire state of California have moved to ban in recent years.

Margarine does edge out butter, but only when selected carefully (and only by a sliver). Because higher levels of trans fat make margarines more solid, you can weed out the trans-fatty options by choosing the varieties that are liquid or sold in tubs. Many varieties now contain water or liquid vegetable oil instead of partially hydrogenated vegetable oil, which can make them virtually free of trans fats.

But the reality is that neither of these spreads can rival olive oil. With butter and margarine, you pick your relative poison; neither is especially good for you. Not so with olive oil. And though most people assume olive oil is simply just not as bad as other fats, it's exceptionally heart healthy.

Here's why. There are two types of cholesterol, one good and the other bad. Good cholesterol is known as high-density lipoprotein, or HDL, and the bad type is referred to as low-density lipoprotein, or LDL. LDL likes to settle cholesterol in your arteries, exactly where you don't want it to be. Both trans and saturated fats raise bad cholesterol and lower good cholesterol, which is exactly the opposite of what you want. Most vegetable oils like corn oil can lower your levels of bad cholesterol, which is nice. But unfortunately they lower your levels of the good kind, too. In the end you don't get much benefit.

Then there is olive oil, the Muhammad Ali of oils: it delivers the magical one-two punch, lowering levels of LDL cholesterol and raising levels of HDL. Olive oil offers other unique benefits as well. It helps prevent free radicals—the scavengers that roam through the body attacking cells and doing damage—from sticking to the walls of your blood vessels. Olive oil is also less likely to congeal and harden in your system, making it less likely to clog your arteries. I've never thought it a coincidence that the person with the world's longest confirmed life span, Jeanne Louise Calment, a Frenchwoman who lived to age 122½, attributed her remarkable longevity to her love of olive oil. She reportedly poured it on all her food and even rubbed it on her skin.

One thing is for sure. Rather than simply add olive oil to your diet in greater quantities, you should use it to replace other fats. In certain recipes where only butter or margarine will do—like some cakes and cookies—a little saturated fat won't exactly kill you. But on salads and in marinades, for example, and at restaurants when you have a choice over what to spread on your bread, always choose olive oil. With those kinds of choices, you never know—maybe one day you'll live to blow out 122 candles, too.

CAN GRAPEFRUIT INCREASE YOUR RISK OF BREAST CANCER?

An e-mail chain that started to jump from inbox to inbox in 2007 had many women fretting. The messages, still floating around, cite an article in the *British Journal of Cancer* that reported an increased risk of breast cancer among postmenopausal women who ate high amounts of grapefruit. In the study, of more than forty-six thousand women overall, those who ate about half a grapefruit every other day had a 30 percent higher risk of breast cancer than those who ate none. The authors said they suspected that several compounds in grapefruit can inhibit an enzyme called CYP 3A4, thus increasing the level of substances that are normally metabolized by the enzyme, including estrogen. Higher levels of estrogen, it's well known, can fuel some types of breast cancer.

Scary stuff.

But perhaps it's time to put this claim to rest. A more extensive follow-up by scientists at Harvard University's public health and medical schools, published in 2008, reached a far different conclusion. That analysis used data from the Nurses' Health Study, which followed more than seventy-seven thousand women, ages thirty to fifty-five, for over a decade. The scientists looked at intake of both grapefruit and grapefruit juice and found no rise in breast cancer risk, either among women overall or among postmenopausal women specifically.

So what to make of the findings? Most experts believe the initial study that started the scare did not account for enough variables and may not have been extensive enough. The verdict is not entirely in yet, but officials at the American Cancer Society say there is not enough evidence for a link to prompt them to change their diet recommendations. No need to throw away the grapefruit—it has too many proven health benefits to ignore—but women who have a family history of estrogen-fueled breast cancer may want to cut back if they're eating grapefruit more than a few times a week.

As Confucius once said, "To go beyond is as wrong as to fall short."

Does mayonnaise make food spoil faster?

Summer is the time of year when food poisoning outbreaks suddenly spike, and there is no picnic ingredient that attracts the suspicious eye of a backyard chef quite like mayonnaise.

Feeling a little nauseous after that Independence Day grill-out? Probably the egg salad. Or maybe it was the potato salad. Or possibly the macaroni salad. Or, well, you get the idea. There are few foods that get as bad a rap as this one.

To some extent it is understandable. A number of large outbreaks of food poisoning at banquets and weddings over the years have been traced to mayonnaise-based salads and foods. But not for the reasons most people might think.

Most brands of commercial mayonnaise, despite their bad rap, contain vinegar and other ingredients that make them quite acidic and, in turn, likely to *protect* you against food poisoning, not subject you to it. When problems occur it is usually the result of one of three things. One is the presence of other contaminated or low-acid ingredients, most commonly chicken, potatoes, and seafood. Another is poor storage or handling—like repeatedly dipping utensils or vegetables and other foods into the mayo—which introduces bacteria to the mix. And the third is the fact that homemade mayonnaise is typically made with unpasteurized eggs, a major source of food-borne illness.

But commercial mayonnaise is another story. The acidic environment is a less than ideal medium for the growth and survival of most bacteria. One group of researchers at the University of

Wisconsin showed this in a classic study by preparing a chicken salad and ham salad in three ways: with commercial mayonnaise, without it, and in the last case with only half the amount recommended in recipes. After contaminating some of the samples with bacteria and then storing them in different conditions for twenty-four hours, the scientists analyzed them again and were surprised by what they found.

When commercial mayonnaise was first added to the salads, the bacteria count either slowed or came to an immediate halt. As the amount of mayo increased, the rate of bacterial growth decreased. And when storage temperatures were raised to those approximating a hot summer day, the growth of bacteria increased in all samples, but the greatest increase was in the samples that did not contain mayonnaise. The mayonnaise, in other words, reduced the odds of spoilage. Who knew?

As for other popular warm-weather picnic foods, there are certainly some to watch out for: meats that are made from the carcasses of many individual animals, like ground beef. According to the Centers for Disease Control and Prevention, a single hamburger can contain meat from hundreds of cows, and all it takes to contaminate it is a pathogen in one animal.

It's also a good idea to be wary of unwashed fruits and vegetables. Top on that list, it turns out, are alfalfa and other raw sprouts, which are often grown in unsanitary, microbe-laden conditions.

So just to recount: Mayonnaise good. Alfalfa sprouts, not always. What'll we find out next—that double bacon cheeseburgers are good for your cholesterol? (One can dream.)

CAN EATING GREEN POTATOES KILL YOU?

It sounds like a joke, or perhaps just an urban legend that grew out of Dr. Seuss's classic *Green Eggs and Ham*. But food scientists say this one is no myth. The reality is that green potatoes contain high levels of a toxin, solanine, which can cause nausea, headaches, and neurological problems.

Potatoes naturally produce small amounts of solanine as a defense against insects, but the levels increase with prolonged exposure to light and warm temperatures. The green color is actually caused by high levels of chlorophyll, which by itself is harmless. But it is also a sign that levels of solanine, which is produced at the same time as chlorophyll, have increased as well.

According to a recent report by Alexander Pavlista, a professor of agronomy and horticulture at the University of Nebraska at Lincoln, a one-hundred-pound person would have to eat about 16 ounces of a fully green potato to get sick. That is the weight of a large baked potato. The report noted that most green potatoes never reach the market. Still, to avoid the development of solanine, it is best to store potatoes in cool, dimly lit areas, and to cut away green areas before eating.

Another good rule: if it tastes bitter, don't eat it. Unlike Dr. Seuss's entree, this green meal would not have a happy ending.

CAN TOO MUCH COLA CAUSE KIDNEY PROBLEMS?

It's well known that too much soda can increase the risk of diabetes and force you to buy new pants with a bigger waist size. But when it comes to kidney problems, is there something about cola that makes it more hazardous than other kinds of soda?

This is the part where a few friends of mine who drink so much cola that they can't go anywhere without bringing their own personal supply would like me to say that the answer is unequivocally no. But unfortunately that is not at all the case.

Colas contain high levels of phosphoric acid, the substance that gives most dark sodas their color and tangy taste but which has also been linked to kidney stones, chronic kidney disease, and other renal problems. Recovering kidney patients in fact are typically told by doctors and nurses to stay away from dark sodas for precisely this reason. But much of this association stemmed from anecdotal and circumstantial evidence, so in 2007 a team of scientists at the National Institutes of Health decided to take a closer look.

Since forcing one group of subjects to drink high amounts of a liquid that's suspected of causing health problems to see what happens is just a tad unethical, the team of scientists conducted what's known as a retrospective study. They recruited 465 people who were newly diagnosed with kidney disease and compared them to 467 healthy people who were matched for age, sex, and race. Then they questioned all the subjects about the types of beverages they typically drank and how often they drank them.

After controlling for various factors, the team found that drinking two or more colas a day—whether artificially sweetened colas or regular ones—more than doubled the risk of kidney disease. And it seems pretty clear that it wasn't the caffeine or the carbonation of the soda that was causing kidney problems, and for this reason: drinking two or more non-cola carbonated drinks a day did not increase the risk. It was cola alone that did the trick.

This may be underscoring the obvious, but it makes sense to limit the number of colas you guzzle in a day. When I spoke to one scientist who has made studying these kinds of associations her life's work, Dale Sandler, the chief of the epidemiology branch at the National Institute of Environmental Health Sciences, she was pretty convinced of what was going on. "There are several epidemiological studies showing the effects of cola on bone mineral density," she said. "The phosphoric acid in the cola may be pulling calcium from the bones, and these higher levels of calcium in the bloodstream can lead to the formation of crystals that lead to kidney stones and other problems."

To be fair, cola is not the only high-phosphate food. Milk, meat, and a few other foods contain high levels of phosphates— but the difference is that they also contain high levels of calcium to balance out the phosphates. Cola, on the other hand, has about as much dietary calcium as this book you're holding in your hands. Nada.

Any doctor worth his or her salt would advise against making cola a regular part of your diet. But in an ABC News article about a woman who developed a twelve-diet-cola-a-day habit, Diana Garza, the communications director of Coca-Cola North America, was quoted with this to say about Diet Coke: "Great taste, no calories, wholesome ingredients. How could you drink too much?" Because what isn't *wholesome* about aspartame, phosphoric acid, carbonated water, and potassium benzoate?

IS A SUGAR RUSH A BETTER PICK-ME-UP THAN CAFFEINE?

The urge to head to bed should typically kick in at some point in the late evening, when darkness falls and the day has come to a close. For me, that urge first kicks in at 2 P.M.

It is always the same. I start my weekdays at 8 or 8:30 A.M. with a light breakfast, then head to work and jump on the story of the day. At noon I find myself in the cafeteria with a knot in my stomach and an overwhelming need for as much food as I can fit on one plate. By 2 P.M. I'm at my desk with my head on my keyboard and my eyes rolling back in my head.

And I know I'm not alone. Millions of Americans are familiar with the post-lunch stupor—or "postprandial sleepiness," in the language of white-coated scientists—which occurs when the spike in blood sugar that follows lunch wears off, inducing the urge to sleep as blood sugar plummets.

Since most workplaces have a policy against napping at, under, or on top of your desk (not that I haven't tried all three), and the method of the artist Salvador Dalí is a tad unorthodox (he was said to work for days on end by taking short, regular naps), turning to a sugary soft drink for a post-lunch energy boost can be incredibly tempting. Forget about caffeine. Sugar, as my thirteen-year-old nephew might say, is where it's at. But is that sugar rush really all it's cracked up to be?

Probably not. The truth is that besides having only short-lasting effects on energy, the sugar high of soft drinks can ultimately work against you, decreasing your attention span, slowing your reaction times, and putting you right back to sleep. It's the well-known phenomenon that even scientists can only describe as crashing.

High sugar content is often taken to mean high energy, but a number of strong studies refute this. In one study, published in the journal *Human Psychopharmacology* in 2006, a group of healthy adults took ninety-minute mental tests after eating a small lunch on various days. On some days, about an hour after lunch, they drank a soft drink that had 42 grams of sugar and about 30 to 40 milligrams of caffeine. On other days, they drank a similarly flavored drink with no sugar or caffeine. With the high-sugar drink, the subjects' test scores were lower and they had more delays in reaction time and lapses in attention. After a fifteen-minute rush of energy, they became tired and less alert. Other studies have found beneficial memory and attention effects for drinks with sugar and caffeine—but only with caffeine levels twice those of a typical soft drink.

All of which means that caffeine is king. But unfortunately most people fail to use it properly. The one or two cups of Colombian or French roast coffee that many people start their days with contain levels of caffeine that even a person running on little sleep—or a longtime coffee drinker with a high tolerance—needs to wake themselves up. According to studies at Harvard Medical School, the best way to consume caffeine is in small, regular doses, like a quarter-cup of coffee every hour, which keeps you alert without increasing the odds of crashing.

Just remember to go easy on the sugar packets.

CAN DRINKING TEA REDUCE STRESS?

This world can be maddening at times.

On some nights when I step outside and stare up at the moon, hanging low like a white peach but still high enough above the Manhattan skyline that I can briefly forget I'm surrounded by gleaming office towers, I'm reminded that it was only a few centuries ago that the typical person lived a life free of technology and the stress and demands that come with it.

Technology is supposed to make our lives easier. But on a normal day, I am stirred awake by a cacophony-spewing alarm clock, herded onto a subway car like I was part of a stock of animals rushing onto Noah's Ark, and then forced to stare at a glowing computer screen for so long—all the while cradling a telephone set between my ear and my shoulder—that by the time I stumble back onto that modern-day metal Ark ten hours later, my vision is clouded with spots and my neck tilts uncontrollably to one side.

And that's only the toll of the physical stress. Statistics show that 40 percent of workers describe their jobs as "very or extremely stressful" and that more than a quarter of workers say a typical day at the office leaves them "burned out." That, in turn, according to the National Institute for Occupational Safety and Health, can increase the risk of psychological disorders, impaired immune function, workplace injuries, cancer, and musculoskeletal disorders.

Ah, the wonders of modern life. Small wonder that many Americans are always looking for a quick and easy way to burn some stress on the road or in the office. But other than drawing a large circle on my desk with the words "Bang head here," I have found few techniques that are reliably cheap (massages these days can cost a fortune) or very convenient (I would advise against practicing either meditation or yoga in your cubicle, which can give your boss the impression that you are either sleeping or unbalanced, even if you're executing a perfect handstand).

The one exception I have found may simply be a warm cup of tea.

Some call it nature's tranquilizer, able to smooth away stress and lift the spirits. And it has had that association virtually since the moment it was introduced about five thousand years ago by Shennong, the ancient emperor and so-called father of Chinese agriculture, who supposedly discovered the drink in an "Isaac Newton" moment of serendipitous genius when some tea leaves blew into a pot of water he was boiling. Shennong went on to claim that regular amounts of tea could aid relaxation and cure a host of ailments. But although the idea of tea as stress-buster dates back millennia, it was only in 2007 that a thorough study finally gave it some credence.

Carried out by epidemiologists at University College London and financed by the British Heart Foundation, it involved seventy-five healthy, nonsmoking adults who were weaned from their normal caffeinated beverages—coffee, tea, soft drinks, and so on—during a four-week "washout" period. Then, during a six-week "treatment" phase, some of the subjects were randomly assigned to receive either four cups a day of black tea or a caffeinated placebo. They were also regularly subjected to stressful "behavioral" tasks that caused spikes in blood pressure, levels of cortisol—the "stress hormone"—heart rate, and other indicators of anxiety and stress.

The results showed that all of the subjects pretty much suffered during these sadistic tests (which, perhaps suspiciously, the researchers did not describe in very much detail). But the tea drinkers showed some substantial differences. They seemed to fare much better on cardiovascular measures. Levels of cortisol, which can wreck the immune system and cause other problems when overproduced, were much lower in the tea group. A mere fifty minutes after the stressful events, the tea group showed a 20 percent decrease in cortisol compared to the placebo group. They also had lower levels of platelet activation—indicating a reduced risk of the vascular obstructions that can set off heart attacks—and they showed "a relative increase in subjective relaxation during the post-task recovery period."

"Black tea may have health benefits in part by aiding stress recovery," the researchers wrote.

Exactly what causes these effects is still being teased out. But it's pretty clear that it has something to do with high levels of a group of antioxidants found in tea known as flavonoids, particularly one called epigallocatechin gallate, or ECGC, which helps arteries relax and is found in black, green, and oolong teas. Many large, randomized studies have found that people who regularly drink several cups of tea a day have lower rates of heart disease. There is also emerging evidence that the habit can lower the risk of diabetes and some cancers, though the research is ongoing and still being debated.

Either way, it's pretty clear that the sedative effects of a few cups of tea a day are beneficial, especially when it comes to combating the side effects of stress. Consider it a sort of insurance policy for your health. And it beats spending eighty bucks a day on back massages. That's my cup of tea.

Do spicy foods boost your metabolism?

If you've ever dumped enough Tabasco sauce on your plate to start a small brushfire in your mouth, or ate a chili pepper so hot it could make the devil sweat, then you know there may be no greater gustatory exercise than a spicy meal with extra kick. But is it true, as has long been held, that spicy foods not only heat you up but also speed up the metabolism?

Over the years, various studies have examined the claim and suggested that certain spices can in fact increase metabolic rate by raising body temperature, though to what extent and for how long is unclear. Capsaicin, the compound that gives red chili pepper its powerful punch, creates the largest bump in heat generation, which helps burn more calories immediately after a meal. Black pepper and ginger have similar effects.

Generally, studies have shown that on average a meal containing a spicy dish, like a bowl of chili, can temporarily increase metabolism by about 8 percent over a person's normal rate, an amount considered fairly negligible. But besides a slight uptick in metabolism, spicy foods may also increase feelings of satiety.

One study by Canadian researchers looked at a group of adult men and found that those who were served hot sauce with appetizers before a meal went on to consume on average about two hundred fewer calories at lunch and in later meals than their peers who did not have anything with capsaicin. The researchers suggested that capsaicin may work as an appetite suppressant. A similar study in 2005 followed twelve men and twelve women over a two-day period in which some were given capsules with small amounts of capsaicin and others were given placebo. They found that the capsaicin increased satiety and reduced fat intake as well as overall caloric consumption.

It's something to keep in mind if you're one of the millions of people looking to trim a few extra calories from your diet, not to mention a little boost to your metabolism. But take heed: spicy foods can also worsen symptoms of ulcers and heartburn. Not that this has stopped many people. In fact, at least one prominent politician is a strong advocate.

In early 2008, Hillary Clinton, who was then running for

president and slugging it out with Barack Obama in the Democratic primaries, gave an unusual answer when NBC's Katie Couric asked Clinton how she stayed fit and energized on the campaign trail. "I eat a lot of hot peppers," she replied. "I for some reason started doing that in 1992, and I swear by it. I think it keeps my metabolism revved up and keeps me healthy."

A move to win over primary voters in pepper-loving Texas? Who knows, but her statement may have encouraged some Democrats—and perhaps even a few Republicans—to pour the Tabasco sauce a bit more *liberally*, you might say, at their next meals.

For the brave few who enjoy incendiary foods simply for the gustatory challenge—a group affectionately known as pepperheads—here are some strange but true facts about capsaicin you probably didn't know:

• Studies in animals show that capsaicin kills some cancer cells by forcing them to commit suicide, also called apoptosis. And you thought spicy food made *you* sweat!

• Technically, you cannot "taste" the heat from a spicy meal, since there is no taste bud for "hot" or "spicy." Capsaicin simply triggers a reaction that the brain perceives as pain, which is why you can perceive the heat from capsaicin on other body parts (the eyes, for example, or the rectum), but you can't perceive true tastes like "sweet" or "bitter" in other body parts. It's believed that taste buds only allow us to perceive a handful of tastes: salty, sweet, bitter, sour, and a fifth one known as umami, found in foods like miso and MSG (monosodium glutamate).

• Unlike mammals, birds are largely immune to the overpowering effects of capsaicin, and will readily eat foods loaded with the compound, since their receptor cells are insensitive to it. Many companies that make bird feed add capsaicin to their product, which keeps squirrels and other mammalian pests from eating it.

• In large enough quantities, capsaicin can be deadly (to mammals).

WILL A SPICY MEAL BEFORE BED RUIN YOUR SLEEP?

A little kick to the palate every now and then can be a boon to your health. But for as long as I've enjoyed eating meals with extra heat, I've been told all along never to indulge before bed, lest I spend the night tossing, turning, and waking up in cold sweats.

There's a lot of diverse reasoning behind the warning. A drop in body temperature near bedtime signals to the body that it's time to go to bed, and some argue that spicy foods blunt this effect, ratcheting up your temperature and making it harder to fall—and remain—asleep. Others say that a spicy meal is simply a burden on your digestive system that has nearly the same disruptive effect on slumber as alcohol (alcohol initially induces sleep, but ultimately disrupts activity in a part of the brain called the thalamus, which subsequently leads to wakefulness and middle-of-the-night insomnia).

Either way, a peculiar claim like this is the sort of wisdom that often turns out to be based on no evidence at all—or, worse, flat out wrong. But this is one claim that we can safely slide into the truth column, because research has shown over the years that a spicy meal at night can in fact lead to poor sleep.

The most direct study to show this was published by a team of Australian researchers in the *International Journal of Psychophysiology*. The scientists recruited a group of young, healthy men and had them consume meals that contained Tabasco sauce and mustard shortly before they turned in on some evenings, and non-spiced, control meals on other evenings.

On the nights that included spicy meals, there were marked changes in the subjects' sleep patterns. They spent less time in both the light phase of sleep, known as Stage 2, and the deep, slow-wave phases of sleep, known as Stages 3 and 4. All of which meant that they experienced less sleep overall and took much longer to drift off when their heads hit the pillows.

In their study, the researchers pointed out that indigestion is an obvious explanation. But they also noted that after eating the spicy meals the subjects did in fact have elevated body temperatures. These higher temperatures were most pronounced during the first sleep cycle, which has been linked in other studies to particularly poor quality of sleep.

But it may not be spicy foods alone. In its literature on sleep disorders, the National Institutes of Health had this to say: "Eating just before going to bed, which raises the body's metabolism and brain activity, may cause nightmares to occur more often."

A little *food* for thought for all those incorrigible late-night munchers out there.

WHAT ABOUT CHOCOLATE— CAN IT DISRUPT SLEEP TOO?

Chocolate may be known to stir affection and awaken the taste buds, but some people wonder whether its stimulating effects may have the unpleasant side effect of keeping them up at night.

Chocolate, as many people know, contains caffeine, but in varying amounts depending on the type. For example, a single, 1.5-ounce Hershey's milk chocolate bar contains 9 milligrams, about three times as much caffeine as a cup of decaffeinated coffee, but a dark chocolate Hershey's candy bar contains far more: about 30 milligrams. That is the same as a cup of instant tea, and slightly less than a typical cup of brewed tea, which contains about 40 milligrams of caffeine.

In other words, a dark chocolate dessert, eaten late enough, might leave you counting plenty of sheep.

Keep in mind that chocolate has other stimulants. One is theobromine, the compound that makes chocolate dangerous to pets like dogs and cats because they metabolize it so slowly. Theobromine increases heart rate, causes sleeplessness, and can be found in chocolate, especially dark chocolate, in small amounts. That is why the National Sleep Foundation advocates avoiding chocolate—along with coffee, tea, and soft drinks—in the hours just before you plan on going to sleep.

But there is an alternative. White chocolate does not contain any theobromine, and little if any caffeine.

IS THERE ANY TRUTH TO THE FRESHMEN 15?

Freshman year of college is when cramming takes on a new meaning. For most people it is the only time in life they will find themselves devouring Kierkegaard and pepperoni pizza with a side of ranch dipping sauce at 3 A.M. on a Tuesday.

Which is why most parents who send their kids off to college worry about them picking up more than knowledge. They also have to worry about them picking up those mysterious, widely feared pounds that quietly stalk every first-year student, the Freshman 15.

And why not? If my first year of college was any indication, then for the average freshman, the unofficial meal plan is atrocious: liquor, dorm slop, and late-night junk food. For most students it's their first time away from home and their first time experiencing inordinate amounts of stress. Comfort food at its most extreme becomes the norm.

But the Freshman 15 is a bit like waking up on the floor of a frat house with no memory of how you got there—many college students fear the mere thought of it, but rarely does it happen. First-year students are likely to gain a little extra weight around the middle, but it's more in the neighborhood of three or four pounds than fifteen, and a small percentage of students actually end up shedding some of their weight.

In 2006, one team of researchers looked at weight and body fat changes in a group of sixty-seven freshmen at Rutgers University. Using digital scales and other instruments, they measured the students at the start of the school year and once again at the end. Overall, the students gained an average of about three pounds and showed an average increase in body fat of 0.7 percent. But some of the students lost weight while others gained it. Among those who got heavier, which included forty-nine of the students, the average increase in weight was seven pounds and the average increase in body fat was 0.9 percent. No one in the study actually gained fifteen pounds.

That seems to be the pattern emerging from the research on freshman year weight gain. Many studies have had similar findings. One in 2008, by researchers at the University of Utah, found that about 50 percent of freshmen gained an average of 2.7 pounds, while 15 percent lost weight. Another in 2006 by scientists at San Jose State found that about 59 percent of freshmen gained three or more pounds, while the rest remained stagnant or shed a pound or two. And others have found that over the course of four years of college, women pack on about two pounds, while men end up lugging around an extra four.

Fifteen pounds seems to be extremely rare. Nonetheless, even an increase of seven pounds, which seemed to be common in the study at Rutgers, is nothing to take lightly. Depending on the body it's slapped on, that can mean a significant spare tire and additional health problems. And it's not that difficult to attain. An extra seven pounds over the course of two semesters can be reached simply by consuming roughly one hundred additional calories a day.

The other problem for students: most do not exercise regularly, and do not get five servings of fruits and vegetables each day.

Continue that habit through graduation and beyond, as many people do, and it can have disastrous long-term consequences. It's no wonder that the average person gains about a pound a year through adulthood.

But there are easy ways to stave off that fate—and the Freshman 5—beginning in college. Students can take simple steps, like stocking their mini fridges with fruits and vegetables instead of processed foods and ice cream, and water and diet drinks instead of sodas and other high-fructose corn syrup–containing beverages. Most students keep a microwave in their dorms, but they should also consider keeping a blender, too. Grab a few bananas, apples, and other fruits from the cafeteria, keep them in the fridge, and in a pinch you can throw them in the blender with a couple other ingredients for a quick smoothie that replaces ice cream *and* helps satisfy the daily requirements for fruits and vitamins.

Some other quick tips? Fill up on water and healthy snacks before attending parties, and limit fried foods to one or two occasions a week. Trying to ignore them completely will be almost impossible over the long run, and besides, it's fine to indulge once in a while. It's overdoing it that quickly fills your frame with fat.

Every first-year student must also contend with the stress of classes, exams, and new social experiences. But one way to cope is with regular exercise. Take your study breaks in the gym or on the track, not at the candy bar in the cafeteria.

In the long run it pays off. Like the knowledge you pick up in class, these healthy habits will stay with you for life.

Is there really such a thing as a runner's high?

Picture yourself sprinting across the African savanna thousands of years ago, in the heat of a desperate hunt for dinner.

Other than some plants and skimpy greens, you haven't had a real meal in three days, and your stomach feels like a wet towel bunched into a ball. Finally spotting a meaty gazelle on the edge of a watering hole, you and your tribal mates took off after it, and now you're hot on its trail. Wooden spear in hand, pangs of hunger gripping your stomach, you are determined to catch your prey and commence your long-awaited feast at last.

But with the lightning-fast ability to sprint a mile in thirty seconds, the gazelle is far faster than you and any of your peers. Speed, however, is not your secret weapon; endurance is. You are built to outrun the gazelle by outlasting it. You, like all humans, are built for precisely this kind of long-distance running—tracking your prey for miles at a time—while the gazelle is not.

The gazelle is the drag-racing car that explodes out of the starting gate with a burst of supercharged speed. But it burns through its fuel and slows a short distance later. You are the stock car that keeps barreling down the track, eventually overtaking the competition.

The human body, it turns out, has numerous adaptations for distance running. You have a ligament that extends from the back of your head down your neck—missing in many other animals—that keeps your head from bobbling back and forth as you run. Your gluteus maximus may seem like just a seat cushion, but it also serves to keep you upright when you run. Your head is streamlined, your mouth designed to take in maximum air, and your legs unusually packed with energy-releasing tendons. You have a built-in cooling system—perspiration—that cools you as the sun beats down on you in the throes of your hunt. Your prey, the gazelle, lacks the ability to sweat, and as you keep after it across the savanna, leaving it no time to stop and rest and cool off in the shade, it eventually overheats and collapses, allowing you to move in for the kill.

But perhaps more than any of these adaptations, there is one in particular that propels you forward and allows you to keep going for miles and miles across those open plains in the torturous midday heat: it is the runner's high.

It is a feeling that many people who have forced themselves to slog through a long and grueling but intensely inspiring run—or any demanding endurance exercise for that matter—know well. Physically exhausted after your punishing feat, you feel as if you should be down on your knees dry heaving uncontrollably, and yet you somehow manage to stand there and marvel at how fantastic you feel, wrapped in a blanket of euphoria.

It is more than a sense of accomplishment; it is an intense emotional high, as if you had taken the world's most addictive drug.

But for decades, many scientists denied that there was anything to this, brushing it off as an exaggeration that could never be directly confirmed by studies. Until very recently, that is. In 2007, a team of scientists got the idea to use PET (positron-emission tomography) scans and newly available compounds that highlight chemical changes in the brain to put the runner's high theory to the test. They recruited ten distance runners, told them they were studying receptors in the brain, and then gave them PET scans before and after two-hour-long runs. They also administered psychological tests that assessed their moods before and after they ran.

What they found was fascinating to anyone who appreciates a good exercise. During their runs, the ten subjects experienced surges in endorphins, the feel-good, opioid-like chemicals that produce feelings of euphoria and emotional relief. The greater the release of endorphins, the greater the elevation in mood. But even more intriguing was that these endorphins were particularly active in the prefrontal and limbic parts of the brain, the seat of emotions that comes into play when people fall in love. That may explain why some people are so emotionally overwhelmed by the runner's high that they can be brought to tears (ahem, with the exception of yours truly).

It also explains why many athletes who suffer an injury during a run or event push through it, only to experience the full brunt of the pain later on. The endorphins soothe the pain so you can finish the task at hand. Nowadays that means finishing the race or rounding all the bases. But thousands of years ago, it meant keeping up the chase, staying on the trail of that speedy gazelle, so you could keep your dinner plans and stave off starvation—then celebrate in grand euphoria and live to see another day.

DOES RUNNING ON A TREADMILL BURN FEWER CALORIES THAN RUNNING ON PAVEMENT?

We know that our bodies evolved into running machines over thousands of years spent chasing our dinners across the sun-drenched African savanna. But for every avid runner nowadays, there is a crucial question that our ancestors never had to face: Pavement or treadmill?

Most runners have a strong preference for one or the other. For some there is the overpowering need to experience the thrill of their feet slamming the pavement, the sun beating down, and a swift wind doing its very best to hold them back. For others the treadmill has its own advantages: It is easier on the knees, gives you some idea of how many calories you're burning, usually has a TV nearby, and you don't have to dodge any cars or unfortunate "surprises" left on the sidewalk by dog owners who are less than considerate.

Personally, I fall into the roadrunner category. Though I'm all for using a treadmill in the winter, I've never been thrilled about the mouse-on-a-wheel feeling that I get while sprinting on a machine in the middle of the summer when I could be out in Central Park instead. But apparently I'm not necessarily in the majority. I have met countless runners who could spend all day on a treadmill but wouldn't think of braving the elements, and judging by the exploding popularity of sports clubs with massive floor space devoted to treadmills and other cardio machines, their ranks are rising.

But is one venue better for your body than the other?

By and large the science shows that running outdoors tends to promote a more intense exercise, mostly due to higher impact and the effects of wind and other variables. A number of studies have shown that in general, outdoor running burns about 5 percent more calories than treadmills do, in part because there is greater wind resistance and no assistance from the treadmill belt, which not only softens your impact but does some of the work by pulling your feet forward. Some studies show, for example, that when adults are allowed to set their own paces on treadmills and on tracks, they move more slowly and with shorter strides when they train on treadmills.

On the other hand, running on a treadmill helps reduce the likelihood of injury, which in turn may allow you to run longer and farther. Studies show that treadmill exercisers suffer fewer stress injuries in the leg. One study published in 2003 in the *British Journal of Sports Medicine*, for example, analyzed a group of runners and found significantly higher rates of bone strain and tension during pavement running than during treadmill running, particularly in the tibia, or shinbone. This increased strain can heighten the risk of stress fractures by more than 50 percent, and the tibia just happens to be one of the most frequently injured parts of the body among runners.

So what can you do to stave off injuries *besides* switching to a treadmill? The answer is, plenty. For one, you should try to run on softer surfaces as often as possible, whether it's dirt, grass, or gravel, even if it means simply getting off the path and running along the grass that lines it. You should also keep in mind that if you typically run several times a week, your running shoes will have a life span of about five to six months. Be sure to replace them at the very least twice a year. You might even consider keeping two pairs of shoes and alternating between them regularly: studies show that after subjecting a pair of shoes to several miles of sole- and cushion-flattening jogging, it takes some time for the shoes to regain their bone-protecting resiliency. Last, consider taking a break every now and then—not from exercise, but from hitting the pavement. It's a good idea once a week to swap out a long jog and replace it with a bike ride or several laps in the swimming pool, both of which are much easier on the joints and give them time to recover.

Treadmill runners may not have to worry as much about their legs, but there are ways to add more intensity to the workout. The best thing to do is to use the incline button on the machine: studies show that running steep hills provides a more intense and efficient workout than jogging on a flat surface or even running up stairs. And hey, once in a blue moon, it may not be such a bad idea to get out in the park and pound some grass. You'll trim some fat while working on your vitamin D intake—something that gym membership will not provide.

CAN STRETCHING BEFORE A WORKOUT PREVENT INJURIES?

There was a time not too long ago when stretching before exercise meant grabbing your legs and ankles and flexing out your muscles before jumping into some physical activity. Nowadays, ask about stretching before exercise and a lot of people assume you want to know whether they flex their fingers before plugging *Guitar Hero* into their video console.

But for those of us who still cling to the old-fashioned notion that exercise requires getting off the couch, the question remains: To stretch, or not to stretch?

Ever since the days in grade school when we were forced to wear school-issued sweats and play dodgeball in gym class, stretching has been ingrained into our heads as an absolute must, a way to prevent injury, reduce soreness, and speed post-exercise recovery. But stretching may not fulfill its promise. Most studies have found that whether it's done before or after a workout, it has little effect on either risk of injury or what is commonly known as delayed-onset muscle soreness, that irritating discomfort that sets in the day after some challenging physical activity.

Numerous studies have reached this conclusion. One of the most recent and extensive reports was published in the *Cochrane Database of Systematic Reviews*. The report reviewed ten randomized studies that looked at the impact of stretching before and after exercise, in repeated sessions and in intervals ranging from forty seconds to ten minutes. The authors concluded that stretching had little or no effect on post-exercise soreness.

Another systematic review, by the Centers for Disease Control and Prevention, was published in the journal *Medicine and Science in Sports and Exercise* in 2004. It looked at multiple studies and found that stretching was not significantly associated with a reduction in injuries. In fact, there is evidence that stretching may actually expose you to a greater likelihood of injury—for a number of reasons. Research has shown that even light stretching can cause damage at the cytoskeletal level and, making matters worse, it increases tolerance to pain, making the stretcher more likely to push him- or herself past the point where pain in the stretched muscle should cause them to stop. Damaging a muscle and then exercising it—potentially too vigorously—can be a recipe for serious injury.

Instead, what seems to have a greater protective effect before intense activity is a light warm-up, which gets blood and oxygen flowing to the muscles and gently prepares them for the upcoming task. Low-impact aerobics and jogging are good warm-up routines. It also helps to ease into an activity by starting off slow and then increasing your speed, intensity, or—in the case of lifting—the weight.

Whatever you do, stay away from those funky school-issued sweats. They may warm you up, but they're not cool.

Is it true the tongue is mapped into four areas of taste?

There's yet another section of high school biology textbooks that needs to be rewritten: the one about the tongue consisting of four areas of taste. You may remember it as the "tongue map"—that colorful illustration that neatly divides the human tongue into sections according to taste receptors. There is the tip of the tongue for sweet, the sides for sour and salty, and the back of the tongue for bitter. But recent studies show that while scientists still have much to learn about receptors, the map, at least, is wrong

What is known is that there are at least five basic tastes: sweet, sour, salty, bitter, and the most recently discovered, umami. This last flavor, which means "savory" in Japanese, can be detected in miso, soy sauce, and other Asian foods, particularly those that contain monosodium glutamate, or MSG. And scientists suspect that there are receptors for other flavors as well.

But when it comes to the familiar map of a tongue, we've had it all wrong. In a study published in the journal *Nature* in 2006, a team of scientists reported that receptors for the basic tastes are found in distinct cells, and that these cells are not localized but spread throughout the tongue.

Still, other studies suggest that some parts of our tongues may be more sensitive to certain flavors, and that there may be differences in the way men and women detect sour, salty, and bitter flavors.

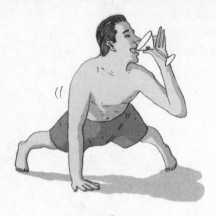

4

DRINK TO YOUR HEALTH

Of Cocktails and Cures

From the gentle euphoria that flows from a glass of perfectly chilled sauvignon blanc, to the deep and dark despair that blankets us on the morning after a shot or two of tequila too many, no other natural substance has brought mankind so many highs and so many lows, so much joy and so much pain, than alcohol.

And no other drug, it seems, has plied mankind with its effects for so long either. Throughout recorded history, alcohol has had a presence in almost every social setting, helping people—and I use the word *help* lightly—engage in everything from celebration to consolation, from romance to relaxation. And like any close acquaintance, it can be soothing in small doses, but turn dreadful when it becomes inescapable.

Love it or hate it, alcohol has had a complicated relationship with humanity that spans thousands of years, going as far back as ancient human history, back to our earliest days on the African savanna, long before civilization sprang forth. Put simply, our history suggests that human beings may be hardwired to enjoy alcohol.

Our early ancestors had a number of adaptations to improve our odds of surviving. We were built with cooling systems that allowed us to outlast the wild animals we chased for days at a time for food. We were given opposable thumbs to allow us to develop weapons and tools. We had taste receptors that seem specifically built for fat, designed to help us get through hard times by seeking out high-density foods. And some scientists believe we also developed a strong predilection for the taste and aroma of alcohol, which made us swoon when we encountered forests and patches of land that were thick with ripe, fermenting fruit—a crucial component in the diets of our distant hunter-gatherer ancestors.

Compared to the sophisticated olfactory systems of other animals, the human sense of smell is blunt and rudimentary. The dog and mouse genomes boast nearly one thousand functional genes for odor receptors, producing a sense of smell that operates like a supercomputer next to the abacus of an olfactory system built from the mere 340 odor receptors in the human genome. But one area where our evolutionary noses excel is alcohol detection. Studies show that primate noses can sniff out alcohol in concentrations that fall below one part per million, and in some cases perhaps even as astoundingly low as ten parts per billion—an olfactory sensitivity for alcohol that rivals even the notorious, super-sniffing capabilities of rodents.

It's not hard to imagine humans putting this ability to use. Stick a glass of a rare and finely aged wine under the nose of a discriminating drinker and she might spend hours dissecting the essence, aroma, and body that overwhelm the olfactory senses. But even the most delicious risotto or succulent cut of lamb, while no doubt pleasing to the palate, cannot elicit quite the same discerning and highly sophisticated response from the human nose.

Anthropologists believe this sensory superpower served us well during our quests for sustenance back in Paleolithic times. If that was the case, then the early human diet contained only low levels of ethanol, since even the ripest fruit generally contains only small amounts. But that too has corollaries today. It may explain the mounds of research showing that low to moderate levels of alcohol are beneficial to health, lowering the risk of heart attack, stroke, metabolic disease, and dementia.

Of course, few of us consume alcohol in the manner in which it seems originally intended. Our Paleolithic ancestors wouldn't recognize all the shots and cocktails and drunken slurring and stammering they'd see if they took a seat at my neighborhood bar on a typical Friday night. Some of us drink alcohol for the flavor, some for the health benefits, and others for the pleasure—or better yet, for all three. We consume it in myriad forms, from miniature glasses of after-dinner port to great big mugs of beer that could dwarf a boot in size and hit the stomach like a loaf of bread.

So let's get to the questions that really matter, the ones that always come up during cocktail hour. Is that rum and cola likely to give you a worse hangover than the vodka cranberries your friends are drinking, and are the calories from that beer you had earlier going straight to your midsection? What about the type of mixer you choose—will that have any effect on how inebriated you get? And for the teetotalers out there, will a glass of grape juice provide the same health benefits as a glass of red? They are made from the same thing, aren't they?

So here we go. A raucous ride through the scientific body of literature on some of alcohol's most intriguing myths and misconceptions. Dive in, and perhaps cradle a glass of your favorite beverage as you flip through the following pages. As Humphrey

Bogart once said, "The problem with the world is that everyone else is a few drinks behind."

DO CALORIES FROM ALCOHOL GO STRAIGHT TO YOUR MIDSECTION?

We know the phenomenon by many names: spare tire, beer belly, beer gut. Some of us know it even better as that round mound of flab that stares back at us in the mirror each morning. But the question is whether there really is something special—or, more likely, loathsome—about the calories in alcohol that make them congregate around our midsections at a greater rate than others.

As tempting as it is to blame the booze for blasting away your abs, that is not quite the case.

In general, drinking causes weight gain primarily because alcohol slows the body's ability to burn fat for energy, not to mention that it increases appetite. The effects of alcohol on the midsection are complicated, but studies show pretty clearly that beer, wine, and spirits have a greater effect on belly fat in adults who drink sporadically than in people who drink regularly but in small amounts. Translation: alcohol in and of itself is not as belly-fattening as most of us tend to think. But drink enough of it, without spreading the drinks out, and, just like any carbohydrate-laden food, it will pack on the pounds.

In one study, published in the *Journal of Nutrition* in 2003, a group of scientists followed more than twenty-three hundred drinkers and nondrinkers and found—after controlling for variables including age, physical activity, and smoking status—that men and women who averaged a single drink per day had the lowest levels of abdominal fat, even lower than teetotalers. Those who drank only occasionally, like once or twice a week, but had four or more drinks in one sitting, had the greatest levels of belly fat. A number of other studies have found the same thing.

One possible explanation is that drinking daily (but in moderate amounts) increases the amount of enzymes that break down alcohol, making regular drinkers better able to digest their drinks. Of course, it also depends on what you choose to accompany those drinks. Beer and bourbon drinkers who subsist on hot dogs and cheese fries will almost certainly sprout a spare tire, while vegan wine sippers might not.

For the most physique-friendly results, drink one or two glasses of liquor a day, about five days a week. It's a regimen that's been shown to help keep the pounds off while cutting the risk of dying from coronary heart disease dramatically. But hold off on it until your later years: studies show this effect only applies to men and women over forty.

Can alcohol warm you up in the winter?

Years ago at a football tailgate held on a winter day that was so frigid I thought I might crack a tooth on my apple cider, I turned to a college buddy of mine and asked him why, in this bitter weather, he was wearing a skimpy cotton shirt and no coat. Lifting his cup of straight whiskey, my friend took a big swig, looked me in the eyes, and calmly said, "Alcohol *is* my winter coat, buddy."

A tough guy, sure. But hard scientific evidence suggests his logic was off. While the right beverage in moderation can bring you some cheer on a chilly winter day, it will not truly warm you up—or at least not for very long. A cup of whiskey or two creates a quick, initial sensation of warmth, but a short time later it decreases core body temperature—regardless of the temperature outside—and increases the risk of hypothermia.

The reason is that the normal process that makes us feel cold takes place when blood flows away from the skin and into the organs, which increases our core body temperature. Drinking alcohol works to reverse this process, increasing the flow of blood to the skin and setting off a sharp drop in body temperature.

It also reverses other reflexes that control body temperature. A study by the Army Research Institute of Environmental Medicine found that the primary mechanism by which alcohol exacerbates the fall in body core temperature is by reducing a person's ability to shiver, which is the human body's way of creating warmth. The more you drink, the faster the slide in temperature. Just how fast, however, depends on the severity of the cold weather and your body composition (the more fat on your frame, the longer it takes to get cold).

Another study, published in 2005, found that after a single drink, the body tries to counteract the brief sensation of warmth caused by increased blood flow to the skin by ramping up its rate of sweating, which only decreases body temperature even further. Making matters worse is that as alcohol lowers body temperature, it also weakens your ability to sense the loss of heat, making you unaware of the problem.

This may not sound like much. But a slew of studies have found that alcohol plays a role in as many as 30 percent of hypothermia-related deaths in some parts of the country. That's a statistic you want to take to heart.

CAN A LITTLE ALCOHOL HELP YOU BEAT A COLD?

It's safe to say that alcohol can cause more calamities than it prevents. After all, there aren't too many other substances that can convince you it's a great idea to start making calls after a night out on the town because your friends—and that ex you broke up with ten months ago—would *love* to hear from you at 4:30

in the morning on a Tuesday. But there may be some exceptions.

When it comes to quick remedies for colds, for example, many people insist that a glass of brandy or a hot toddy—a couple of shots of whiskey mixed with hot water and lemon juice—is just what the doctor ordered.

The Irish and the Scots have been dispensing hot toddies to sniffling cold sufferers for ages, and I can attest that during a trip to Dublin a few years ago to seek out some of my ancestors, I noticed that the hot toddy is still very much a part of the standard medicine kit. I suffered a cold on exactly two occasions, and overall had no less than ten people offer me their personalized hot toddy recipes. Then again, this is also a country where alcohol is widely dubbed an essential food group. Let's also not forget that the word *whiskey* derives from the Gaelic word for water, *uisce* or *uisg*, and that in its Gaelic entirety, *uisce beatha*, it means "water of life."

Water equals whiskey? Only on the Emerald Isle.

It's not all that difficult to see how mild inebriation can have the potential to relieve cold and flu symptoms, but so far no study has shown that alcohol has the ability to kill germs in the bloodstream or stop a cold in its tracks. And while alcohol may provide temporary relief by clearing the sinuses and eventually inducing sleep, there is also the small risk of it prolonging symptoms by increasing dehydration. The American Lung Association, for example, advises steering clear of alcohol and caffeine during a cold for precisely that reason.

Nonetheless, two large studies have found that although moderate drinking may not exactly cure colds, it can help keep them at bay. One study, by researchers at Carnegie Mellon University in 1993, involved 391 adults split into two groups: one that received a benign saline solution, and another group of brave subjects who were each exposed to one of five respiratory viruses. Ultimately what this study demonstrated—other than the willingness of scientists to put their subjects through the ringer—was that resistance to colds increased with moderate drinking, *except* in smokers. People who sipped up to three or four drinks a day were far less likely to develop colds than their peers.

Then, in 2002, researchers in Spain followed forty-three hundred healthy adults and examined their habits and susceptibility to colds. They did not find much of a relationship between consumption of spirits and susceptibility to colds, but they did show that drinking eight to fourteen glasses of wine, particularly red wine, per week was linked to as much as a 60 percent reduction in the risk of developing a cold. It seems that red wine may be particularly effective in this scenario because of its antioxidant properties.

Thus, you can go with a hot toddy and find some comfort in a glass when you're feeling under the weather, but keep in mind that you run the risk of dehydration. At least be sure to add some other liquids to that regimen. But it's also a far better idea to bulk up your immunity with the occasional cocktail or daily glass of wine to keep those colds from showing up in the first place.

As Benjamin Franklin once said, "Alcohol is proof that God loves us and wants us to be happy"—or in this case healthy.

Anahad's hot toddy recipe, culled from primary research in Ireland:

1 pint of water
Zest of ½ lemon, plus juice of ½ lemon
1 tablespoon of fresh mint leaves
3 or more teaspoons of brown sugar
2 or more generous shots of whiskey

Add all the ingredients to a pot except the lemon juice. Heat to a boil. Add the lemon juice.

DO YOU GET DRUNK FASTER WHEN YOU DRINK AT HIGHER ALTITUDES?

At the 2008 Democratic convention in the mile-high city of Denver, the New York State Democratic Party included in its information packet for delegates a strong warning about the effects of alcohol at high altitudes. "Please monitor yourself, and remember that drinks may go to your head faster than you're used to," it said. "We don't want any of our members to miss Delegation events or proceedings, so please stay safe."

Coloradoans like to boast that one drink in the mountains is twice as potent as it would be anywhere else, and even the Denver visitors bureau advises out-of-towners to go easy on the Rocky Mountain brew. It's the reason many hikers insist on keeping their climbs alcohol free, and the reason flight attendants and other airline employees like to limit the flow of liquor—not to mention boarding passengers who are already intoxicated—on most flights.

An old and oft-repeated saying, it is based on the notion that lower oxygen levels at high altitudes impair the ability to metabolize alcohol, leading to quicker absorption and greatly enhanced intoxication. But call it a tale of tall proportions: studies have found that alcohol is no more potent at high altitudes than it is at sea level.

First, there's the metabolic argument. Alcohol is metabolized by an enzyme called alcohol dehydrogenase, which converts the substance to a harmless by-product, acetaldehyde. But this reaction doesn't require any catalytic assistance from oxygen, so the notion that lower oxygen levels might hamper it does not hold up. Then there are those who say it's simply the greater barometric pressure at high elevations that enhances inebriation—higher levels of pressure mean alcohol is absorbed into the bloodstream more quickly.

But years of research have failed to bear those theories out.

In a series of studies by the Federal Aviation Administration, scientists used pressure chambers to simulate the effects of high altitude, and performed blood alcohol tests on groups of subjects who drank under ground-level and high-altitude conditions. There was no difference between the two.

In other studies, scientists examined people at altitudes of 12,000 feet and higher and found that the altitude alone—without alcohol—could induce a state of fatigue that hampers mental and physical abilities. When the subjects were given a battery of cognitive tests, they earned lower scores under the high-altitude conditions than at ground level.

When they were given four drinks at sea level, however, they also did worse—significantly worse, in fact, than they did at high altitude. Considering what happened under the two separate conditions, you would think that combining them would produce a synergistic effect that lowered scores dramatically. But that was not the case at all. Having the subjects consume four drinks under conditions of high elevation had only a slightly greater impact on cognitive performance than the four drinks alone, suggesting that altitude was not "enhancing" the alcohol, but having its own small, separate effect.

In the end, the added effect of the altitude on top of four drinks was the equivalent of taking another sip or two. In other words, it was the equivalent of not much at all.

What we can say for sure is that the air in Colorado is thin. But your tolerance—well, despite what the locals may tell you, maybe not so much.

CAN SOME MIXERS MAKE YOU MORE DRUNK?

Usually it is the liquor component of a cocktail—not the mixer—that we all look to when considering a drink's inebriating abilities. We grab a bottle and splash some in our already filled glasses, concerned only about that final, fleeting dose of sweet, sour, or savor. It is forgotten as soon as it crosses the threshold of our taste buds and the liquor slowly starts to work its way into our bloodstream. Whether seltzer water or sour mix, cranberry juice or cola, the cocktail mixer is the much-needed mask that makes the unpleasant pleasant—the adult equivalent of the added fruit flavor that keeps the cough syrup down. The mixer is the afterthought.

But the time has come to give the almighty mixer its proper due, for it acts far more synergistically with alcohol during the inebriation process than most of us ever imagined. Depending on the beverage chosen, the mixer can speed or slow your rate of intoxication and heighten or lower your peak blood alcohol concentration.

A good example of this is the way alcohol acts differently when mixed with either diet or nondiet juice and soda. Diet drinks seem to enhance the effects of alcohol, making it kick in faster and last longer. A study published in the *American Journal of Medicine* demonstrated this directly. In it, a team of scientists recruited a group of healthy subjects and had them consume vodka cocktails on different occasions. On some occasions, the subjects drank a 20-ounce drink mixed with a sugar-sweetened beverage, and on others they drank a 20-ounce cocktail that was identical in every respect except that it was mixed with an artificially sweetened diet beverage. On the occasions when the subjects drank the cocktails mixed with the diet drinks, the alcohol entered their bloodstreams at a rate that was an astonishing fifteen minutes faster than the rate at which it was absorbed when mixed with the sugar-sweetened mixer. And that wasn't it: with the diet drinks, the subjects' blood alcohol concentrations climbed higher, peaking at 0.05 percent, compared to only 0.03 percent with the regular mixer.

So what happened?

It turns out that alcohol is absorbed more quickly when

there is no sugar to slow it down, which means that artificial sweetener—which essentially passes straight through our systems unaltered—does nothing to hold back alcohol. It allows it to pass through our stomachs quickly and slip straight into the bloodstream. There is very little additional digestive activity—like the breakdown of sucrose, as with nondiet drinks—to slow it down. This goes not just for diet drinks, but also for tap water, seltzer water, and any other drink that does not contain sugar.

But that's not all. There is also the way alcohol acts differently when mixed with carbonated or noncarbonated drinks. Carbonation speeds up the rate at which alcohol is absorbed, which is why that first sip of champagne every New Year's Eve goes straight to your head. A 2007 study that compared the difference between flat and carbonated drinks in a group of people showed that when mixed with fizzy drinks, alcohol enters the bloodstream almost four minutes faster, which can certainly make you feel a lot drunker.

All things considered, seltzer water, with its lack of sugar and its inebriation-inducing effervescence, will be most likely to enhance the effects of a cocktail. Better to opt for something flat and slightly more substantial, like orange and cranberry juice or low-sugar margarita mixes. But either way, any mixer is better than no mixer, particularly when it comes to those of us who prefer tequila over table wine.

CAN SOME TYPES OF ALCOHOL CAUSE WORSE HANGOVERS THAN OTHERS?

We all know that too much alcohol of any kind can cause sickness and regret the morning after—and, for the unlucky few, a stomach-clearing trip to the porcelain throne. But it's often said that some kinds of drinks can make that dreaded morning-after a lot less dreadful, and others, well, let's just say a lot more painful.

I personally have always been told that red wine produces the worst hangovers, which helps to explain why I've developed my predilection for sauvignon blanc. And it turns out that was not a bad idea. Research shows that the type of alcohol you drink can in fact make a difference, though for various reasons. Among the most important is the amount of congeners (pronounced CON-juh-nurz) found in your drink. These complex organic molecules are a by-product of the fermentation process, and they are the culprits that make those who imbibe just a little too much feel sorry about it the next day. Impurities in poorly refined spirits, like cheap vodka, can also play a role, but congeners, which are common in darker liquors, seem to have the greatest effect.

According to one report in the *British Medical Journal*, which looked at the effects of different types of alcohol on a large group of volunteers, the drink that produced the most hangover symptoms was brandy, followed by red wine, rum, whiskey, white wine, gin, and vodka. "Vodka and pure ethanol," the report stated, "caused only mild headaches in two volunteers." Another study showed that drinking bourbon was twice as likely to cause sickness as drinking the same amount of vodka.

There is also wide variation within certain categories, like wine. Wines that come from countries where a small change in climate can greatly affect their quality, for example, can contain significantly more hangover-inducing compounds in a bad season. And cheaper, lower-end red wines in particular are known to contain high levels of congeners.

The take-away message here is that if you have somewhere to be the morning after a big night out on the town, you're generally better off going with vodka sodas over Jack and colas, with some water in between your drinks to speed up the removal of congeners from your system. That'll surely reduce the severity of any hangover.

But all of this raises a pressing question for those of us who would prefer to enjoy a glass of whiskey or two (or three) and not worry about a hangover at all: If alcohol has been around for thousands of years, and we know exactly why it causes hangovers, then why has a true hangover cure remained so elusive?

ARE THERE ANY PROVEN HANGOVER CURES?

There are some topics of research that even scientists are afraid to touch.

Take a good look at the medical literature on alcohol, and you'll see that scientists are more concerned with studying alcohol dependence than alcohol-induced hangovers. That's why even the most popular and widely touted remedies have no legitimate studies backing them up—because that kind of research is widely considered unethical. The quiet truth is that there aren't many scientists who want their claim to fame to be that they made it possible for school bus drivers to go out, get drunk, and then wake up and pop a pill so they can drive your kids to school.

But a few brave scientists took the bold step of looking beyond that worst-case scenario so they could help those of us who would simply like, on occasion, to enjoy a long night of partying and still wake up feeling refreshed. Dogs may be a man's best friend, but anything that can cure or prevent a hangover would definitely be his most *useful* friend. So here's a review of the winners and losers among some popular hangover remedies.

First up is one that has endured through the ages, despite the fact that it's not considered effective: black coffee. Its hangover cure status probably came about because caffeine is a vasoconstrictor, which reduces the size of blood vessels, and can help alleviate some headaches. Unfortunately, hangovers are caused by dehydration, and caffeine is a diuretic, meaning it increases water loss. That could lead to even more dehydration.

Then there's the other breakfast-themed remedy, burnt toast. This one supposedly works because the carbon in the charred bread works like charcoal, soaking up the alcohol and its by-products. Charcoal, which also contains carbon, is an age-old treatment for many severe poisonings, like drug overdoses. The problem, however, is that the carbon in burnt toast is not the same as the kind in activated charcoal. And activated charcoal isn't used to treat alcohol poisoning anyway.

On to a tastier remedy: fruit juice. The nutrients fructose and glucose in fruit juices are said to reduce the fatigue brought on by a hangover and remove some of the toxic by-products. Unfortunately, a study of more than one hundred healthy volunteers found that such beverages had little or no effect on the intensity of alcohol intoxication and hangover—whether they were consumed while drinking or the next morning.

A little hair of the dog that bit you? This phrase stems from an old belief that the way to prevent rabies after a dog bite was to literally get some hair from the dog that bit you, and then rub it into the wound. Unfortunately, relieving a hangover with more alcohol has the same effect as rubbing dog hair in a wound: it only makes things worse. That's because while more alcohol can stave off the hangover—it helps relieve the withdrawal symptoms that are partly responsible for the pain—it cannot completely eliminate it. It just delays it, and makes it fiercer. Sooner or later, the hangover is going to strike, and the body will only have more toxins to process—meaning plenty more pain.

What about all those over-the-counter hangover pills? Many of them are bunk, and some are even made by the same companies that hawk "penis enhancement" pills on late-night television. But according to Hangover Review, an independent Web site that conducted studies of many of the hangover pills, a few actually work. The site gave a thumbs-up to Sob'r-K Hangover Stopper, Uncle Rummie's Hangover Helper, and Chaser—all of which use carbon. But it's really no surprise that some of these products are effective. Most of them require taking them with a full glass of water, and then taking more throughout the evening with—guess what—more water. Perhaps it's the *water*, not the pills, that's helping to relieve the pain? You could replace the pills with breath mints, and as long as you were taking them with water, you'd still reduce the severity of any hangover.

Or how about eating a big, heavy meal? Plenty of people say that a large meal before you finally call it a night will bust any hangover, mostly because the food soaks up the booze. I know I've certainly been tempted to follow this rule over the years, and I've eaten so much late-night, post-drink pizza that I can't have a slice without getting an urge for a beer. Fortunately, a team of Swedish scientists put this maxim to the test. They found that it works, but up to a point. When men and women drank roughly 50 grams of alcohol—the equivalent of either four beers, three glasses of red wine, or three cocktails—and consumed a meal, they reported nothing more than mild hangover symptoms the next morning. But the meal made no difference for subjects who drank 80 grams of alcohol, the equivalent of roughly six beers, about five glasses of wine, or roughly five mixed drinks. Most of them woke up with raging hangovers. "The most common symptoms were headache, drowsiness, and fatigue," the scientists reported. But take it from me: a hangover is bad enough, but a hangover on a full stomach is even worse. It's the reason I switched from a slice of pizza before bed to a giant glass of water and two ibuprofen.

If you are going to count on food, you might try something with eggs. They're high in cysteine, a substance that helps counter the effects of acetaldehyde, the alcohol by-product that causes many of the symptoms of a hangover. There haven't been any studies that looked directly at whether eating eggs can ease a hangover, but limited research in animals suggests it might.

One technique you may have heard and ignored is taking vitamin B_6. Surprisingly, it may actually work. In one study, scientists had men and women attend two parties and drink until they were intoxicated. One group of subjects received 1,200 milligrams of B_6 that was split into three doses: 400 milligrams at the start of the party, 400 milligrams three hours later, and the rest at the end of the night. The other group, which attended the other party, received placebos. Neither group knew for sure what they were getting. Turns out that the B_6 group had half the hangover symptoms of the placebo group. That's not bad. But keep in mind that B_6 in high doses can cause severe side effects, like nerve damage and other neurological problems. It's not clear what an occasional dose of 1,200 milligrams might do, but studies show that daily doses of 1,000 milligrams or more can cause sensory neuropathy.

It seems that nothing is quite perfect, except more water and less alcohol. Hangovers have been reported since biblical times, and odds are they'll continue plaguing us for centuries to come. As one study of hangovers points out, it is a sentiment summed up nicely by George Ade in his 1903 musical comedy, *The Sultan of Sulu*:

R-E-M-O-R-S-E!
Those dry Martinis did the work for me:
Last night at twelve I felt immense,
Today I feel like thirty cents.
My eyes are blurred, my coppers hot,
I'll try to eat, but I cannot.
It is no time for mirth and laughter,
The cold, gray dawn of the morning after.

DOES GRAPE JUICE HAVE
THE SAME HEALTH BENEFITS
AS RED WINE?

By now the cardiovascular benefits of a daily glass of red wine or two are well known. But in the wake of all the research touting the heart-healthy rewards that wine can offer, many tee-totalers had an obvious question that was drowned out by all the fuss: Can we reap the same nutritional bonanza from wine's un-fermented sibling, or are we locked out of the party?

With much pleasure I can offer this news: Grape juice may not provide much of a buzz, but when it comes to its ability to avert heart disease, you can still toast to good health.

Alcohol itself, in moderation, can relax blood vessels and in-crease your levels of the good, or HDL, cholesterol. But the substances that provide much of red wine's cardioprotective effects—resveratrol and the antioxidants called flavonoids—are also found in grape juice, especially the varieties made from red and dark purple Concord grapes. Red grapes are high in two flavonoids—quercetin and rutin—that are especially potent and, unfortunately, absent in white grapes.

A number of independent studies have found that like alcohol, grape juice can reduce the risk of blood clots and prevent LDL, or bad, cholesterol from sticking to coronary arteries, among other cardiac benefits. One study, conducted by scientists at the Univer-sity of Wisconsin, looked at the effects of two servings of Concord grape juice a day in fifteen people with coronary artery disease. Af-ter two weeks, the subjects had improved blood flow and reduced oxidation of LDL cholesterol (oxidized LDL cholesterol can dam-age arteries and lead to blockages).

Other studies in humans and some animals, including one published in 2007 in the journal *Atherosclerosis*, have shown that daily consumption might lower blood pressure and cholesterol levels. Beware that some varieties of grape juice are loaded with sugar and artificial ingredients. Many stores carry natural varieties, which means you'll be able to get all the heart-healthy benefits of red wine without too much sugar—and even after two or three glasses, you'll still be able to drive.

CAN A SILVER SPOON IN A BOTTLE OF CHAMPAGNE KEEP IT FROM GOING FLAT?

It's an old tradition, started by the French (naturally) as a way to keep every champagne-fueled New Year's Eve party going as long as possible—that is, by keeping the champagne from going flat for hours, and even days, after the cork is popped.

The method is simple. Grab a silver spoon, stick it in the neck of the unfinished bottle of bubbly so that the spoon is hanging handle down, and slide the bottle in the refrigerator. When the bottle is retrieved and the remaining champagne poured, it should still have its tongue-tingling sparkle.

Unfortunately, this bit of old French folklore is flawed. A chemistry professor at Stanford University decided to put the claim to the test after a German reporter called him to ask whether it was true. In his study, the chemist, Richard Zare, convened a panel of eight taste-testers. Then he had the subjects taste and score ten different bottles of champagne, all of which had their labels covered and were kept at perfect temperature. There were five different conditions. In one, the bottle was opened just before the test. In another, it was opened and left uncorked for twenty-six hours. In a third it was kept open for about a day, with either silver or stainless steel spoons dangling in the neck. And in the last the bottle was opened and then recorked and refrigerated.

After several rounds of tasting, they found that the spoons not only failed to keep the champagne sparkling, but surprisingly only seemed to accelerate the flattening. Even more surprising was that the worst method of all was recorking—it caused the champagne to lose taste and flatten the most. The best method, it turned out, was simply leaving the bottle open in the refrigerator. The study could not explain why that is, though. It seems that each bottle is its own little microenvironment, and the factors contributing to the loss of the carbon dioxide that gives champagne its effervescence can vary from one bottle to the next.

And of course, you can always try my method for handling an open bottle of champagne: finish the thing!

IS NEW YEAR'S THE MOST DANGEROUS TIME TO BE ON THE ROAD?

Could the most celebratory day of the year also be the most dangerous for drivers?

With all the open bars, people on the road, and rejoicing in the streets, it is easy to imagine that New Year's is a risky time. Holidays in general are the most hazardous time for drivers, a result of sharp increases in traveling and drunken driving. And when it comes to New Year's, research over the years offers sobering statistics.

But according to research by the Insurance Institute for Highway Safety, which examined accident data in the United States from 1986 to 2002, the day of the year with the most fatalities from accidents is the Fourth of July, with an average of 161. Not far behind are July 3 (149) and December 23 (145). New Year's Day is fourth, with 142.

A closer look, however, reveals something peculiar: New Year's Day is the deadliest for pedestrians. In the study period, 410 of those killed on New Year's were pedestrians, slightly more than on Halloween (401). For New Year's, the problem was largely that of increased drinking and celebrations. Half the deaths involved alcohol impairment, and 58 percent of the pedestrians who were killed had a high blood-alcohol concentration, the study found.

Something to keep in mind as the champagne starts to flow next December 31.

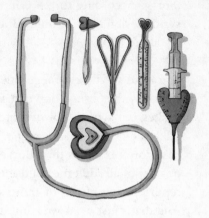

5
LOVE MEDICINE
And Other Bedroom Matters

For most people, the only time we are not consumed by the pursuit of sex—consciously or otherwise—is when we are in the middle of the act itself.

As a health reporter, this I know for certain.

I am often amazed by the volume of sex-related questions I am asked to investigate—many of them so unusual they had never crossed my mind. Based on the contents of my in-box, somewhere out in America at this very moment, someone is wondering to what extent tongue size correlates to sexual prowess. In another town not far away, someone else would love to know whether condoms are just as effective when used in a hot tub. (Studies say? Not a good idea. Take the party inside.) And on another coast, a person is dying to know whether she can lower her risk of sexually transmitted diseases (STDs) if she immediately urinates after sex.

(Sorry: According to the Centers for Disease Control and Prevention, don't count on it. But it's always good to exercise the bladder.)

Over the years, as I've sought out answers in the medical literature to these strange queries and many others, I've been struck by the observation that so much of human behavior—our desires, our actions, how we interact with one another—is permeated by hidden sexual meaning. This, of course, is in a nation that has more sex shops than Burger Kings, and a nation in which a quarter of all adult men and about 10 percent of all adult women report having fifteen or more sexual partners in their lifetimes. And that's just what we admit to. As a friend of mine is fond of saying, whatever a woman says her number is, multiply that by two to get the true figure. For a man's true number, take the figure he gave you and subtract five.

Either way, our attitudes toward sex reflect a simple thing: the more chaste and sexually repressed a society is, the more that society seems to become obsessed with sex. In other countries—including Sweden, Germany, Denmark, and Japan—scientists have found that as restrictions on access to pornography are relaxed, the rates of sex offenses take surprising turns downward. Studies in the United States have found similar drops in sex offenses when Internet access is increased (interestingly, the effect applies only to sex offenses and not to other serious crimes, like homicide). In other words, if you douse the forest with water, you're less likely to see a brushfire.

Other countries have long led the United States on the road toward sexual openness. It was not that long ago that major American universities were single-sex only, couples on television shows like *I Love Lucy* could not be shown in bed together, and even mentioning the word *orgasm* was considered taboo. Some of that squeamishness is still alive. As a health reporter at an institution known for its professorial tone, I have occasionally come up against a few taboos myself. In one column on whether oysters are an aphrodisiac, I wrote that ancient cultures connected the oyster to sex because they found its "shape and texture" reminiscent of female genitalia. "Whoa," an editor remarked, deleting the line. "That's *way* too graphic. Let's remember that this is a family paper."

Veteran health reporters joke all the time about being the first to introduce seemingly innocuous medical terms into the paper—like *clitoris* and *labia*—after numerous face-offs with the standards editors. They wear these sexual-groundbreaking badges proudly. But unlike my trailblazing colleagues, I see no need to break new ground by introducing any previously unpublishable language into the *Times* vernacular.

However, in the spirit of sexual freedom, here's a chance to explore some of the most popular sexual quandaries that haven't yet made it into the newspaper. It's time to shake off our sexual squeamishness and throw back the cover on some tantalizing bedroom matters.

CAN SEX BE SUBSTITUTED FOR A WORKOUT?

Sexercise, anyone?

Sex can definitely be considered a good cardiovascular workout. But unless your idea of sex involves swinging from the chandeliers or using your partner to do bench presses, you probably won't burn enough calories to forgo other forms of exercise.

Let's do the math. According to the National Center for Health Statistics, the average weight for an adult man is 190 pounds, about 30 pounds more than the average weight of an adult woman, 162 pounds. Based on data collected in the *Compendium of Physical Activities*, the average man burns about fifty-three calories during thirty minutes of moderate sexual activity, and the average woman burns about forty-four calories.

Ah, but you're a virile, athletic, and hot-blooded sexual machine, you say, and the words *moderate* and *brief* in no way accurately describe what you're capable of. Okay, point taken. So let's consider an hour of vigorous sexual activity. That means for the average man burning 122 calories and for the average woman burning 102 calories.

That's not bad at all. But let's compare that to some other physical activities. The average man, meanwhile, expends 245 calories during an hour of moderate weight-lifting, which includes free weights and machines; the average woman burns about 255 calories an hour doing Pilates. Here are the figures for some other activities, performed over an hour, for comparison's sake:

Jogging on a treadmill at five miles an hour: 702 calories for men, 585 calories for women

Stationary bicycling, at a moderate pace: 572 calories for men, 508 calories for women

Performing low-impact aerobics: 431 calories for men, 340 calories for women

Playing catch: 204 calories for men, 181 calories for women

Brushing your teeth (not that anyone would ever spend an hour doing this): 163 calories for men, 145 calories for women

Tango dancing: 259 calories for men, 204 calories for women

Dressing and undressing: 172 calories for men, 136 calories for women

Skiing downhill, at a moderate pace: 517 calories for men, 408 calories for women

As you can see, an hour of Pilates beats out an hour of vigorous sex when it comes to basic energy expenditure.

But all of these activities, besides simply burning calories, target different muscles and areas of the body, providing unique workouts. Sex, for example, helps strengthen your abs, hamstrings, and quadriceps, while aerobics and jogging target a variety of muscles in their own ways. Sex also has some other unique benefits. Research over the years suggests it may reduce stress, strengthen the immune system, and even boost longevity. In other words, a little sexual activity isn't exactly enough to replace the local gym, but it might go a long way toward improving your health.

Not that you necessarily needed any incentives in the bedroom.

DO SHORT MEN HAVE LESS LUCK WITH WOMEN?

Short men get the shortest shrift.

Women may be loath to admit it, but deep down, the great majority seem to harbor a strong reluctance to dating short men—that is, men who fall below the average adult height, five foot nine inches.

How do I know this? One: because I see how much my vertically challenged friends struggle in the dating department. Sure, some women will insist that height doesn't matter—it's what you do with it that counts. Intelligence, ambition, confidence, style, good looks, and a sense of humor will make up for any, ahem, shortcomings in the height department, they say. Look no further than Prince, Tom Cruise, Frank Sinatra, and Bono, and at other successful men who could easily shop in the boy's department and yet seem to have no problem snagging beautiful women, right?

Consider those men outliers. In addition to my personal observations, years of scientific research has revealed ample evidence that short men suffer from romantic discrimination. Take, for example, a study published in 2005, brought to us by a team of randy anthropologists who studied the traits that women in heat look for in men. They found that women more often look for taller males, but that this is especially the case when they're in the follicular—or most fertile—phase of their menstrual cycles. That was a sign that women, whether they were consciously aware of it or not, were selecting the genes of taller males for their offspring. And the effect was seen in women regardless of whether they themselves were tall or short.

Other studies have shown that taller men have more female partners and more active dating lives. By all indications, when compared to shorter men, taller men seem to win out, even when it comes to reproductive success. One large study in 2002 that followed a cohort of adult men, looking at their relationships with women, found that men who were taller were more likely to find a long-term partner, more likely to have several different long-term partners, and less likely to be childless than their shorter counterparts. They were also more likely to have high socioeconomic status. The study put it bluntly. "This confirms the finding that tall men are considered more attractive and suggests that, in a noncontracepting environment," or, in other words, a society where birth control pills and other contraceptives aren't available, "they would have more children."

"The conclusion," the study went on, "is that male tallness has been selected for in recent human evolution."

But perk up, short men of the world. The news is not all bad. There are some advantages to being closer to the ground—and more compact. Shorter men are less likely to die in car crashes, break bones in a fall, or suffer serious injuries, and they have lower rates of some diseases (in part because reaching a greater height means your cells have to replicate and duplicate more frequently, opening the door to more wear and tear and oxidative damage).

Now if only women could be persuaded to find these traits more attractive . . .

Can being on birth control increase your chances of becoming infertile?

The birth control pill may simplify life for a lot of women, but in an age when even the seemingly harmless medications can have unpleasant side effects, it's natural to wonder whether taking the pill long-term may have serious consequences. It may be small, and convenient, but the big task of the little pill is to essentially manipulate the reproductive system, preventing ovulation. What's to say that once this process is suppressed long enough—repeatedly, over years and years—it does not simply shut off altogether, leaving a woman infertile? Or might it, at the very least, reduce a woman's fertility?

The reality is that the pill, even after years of use, won't increase your chances of becoming infertile. But for women who use it for a while, stop it, and try to become pregnant, it may increase the time it takes to reach success.

One reason is that the pill can reduce levels of the cervical fluid that facilitates pregnancy by allowing sperm to swim through the cervix and reach a woman's egg. Often, once the pill is stopped, the cells that produce this fluid regenerate, returning things to normal. When that doesn't happen, the woman has other options, like intrauterine insemination. But even when the cells that produce cervical fluid regenerate, it may take some time for pregnancy to occur.

Take a study published in 2001 that followed nearly eleven hundred women between the ages of eighteen and forty—none of whom had previously given birth—for about a decade. Over the course of the study, the scientists looked at the differences between those who used condoms, intrauterine devices, or oral contraceptive, trying to figure out what happened when the women who eventually decided they were ready to get pregnant stopped their contraception of choice and gave it a shot. What they found was that 54 percent of the women who had been using condoms delivered a baby within a year of trying. For other methods, the success rate was lower. About 39 percent of women who had been using intrauterine devices delivered within a year, compared to 32 percent of those who had been taking the pill. You may be wondering why the women using intrauterine devices had an increased time-to-pregnancy as well. Scientists suspect it may have something to do with the IUD increasing the risk of a woman developing pelvic inflammatory disease, perhaps because inserting the device can introduce bacteria into the uterus, setting off infection.

Boy, the things women endure that men are spared from having to experience. Nine months of labor, monthly periods, and birth control pills. If you're a woman, you must be waiting for the day when men get to know what it's like, or at least remove some of the burden from your shoulders. Well, that day may now be in the offing . . .

WILL THERE EVER BE A MALE BIRTH CONTROL PILL?

Here's a scenario. Imagine walking into a gritty sports bar and taking a seat at the bar next to two men watching a football game over some beers. One of the men takes a swig, turns to his buddy, and raises a question.

"Hey bro, you take your birth control today?"

It's hard to envision. But it might one day be the norm.

That is, of course, once scientists produce the first male birth control pill, which is very much in their sights. Whether men will actually take it is another question, but it is likely that one will be on the market in roughly 2015.

The first clinical trials involving a male contraceptive began in 2001, and since then scientists have managed some success. Several different methods have been studied—a patch, an injection given once every few months, a gel, a pill, and an implant inserted under the skin—but as of 2008 none had been perfected. Most have been able to hamper sperm production in men, the ultimate objective, but all seem to have a failure rate of at least 5 percent.

The problem is that men produce hundreds of millions of sperm, and the little buggers are far more difficult to suppress than the single egg produced each month by a typical woman. And the sperm-blocking effects of any male contraceptive must be reversible; otherwise it would essentially make its users permanently sterile.

One method of doing this is by creating a hormonally based pill that includes testosterone. In general, after the testes produce sperm, they release testosterone into the bloodstream along with another hormone, called inhibin, which alert the brain that production is complete. Eventually, when the sperm is depleted, that process starts over. But if testosterone is already circulating in the blood in high enough levels—thanks to a pill—then the brain is led to believe that the body has enough sperm. The only problem is that taking testosterone produces side effects similar to those seen in steroid abusers, like acne and liver problems.

As a result, scientists have sought to create a pill that also includes progestogen, another hormone that helps suppress sperm production and can offset some of the problems associated with a testosterone pill. But progestogen has some side effects of its own.

Most of the other methods involve some combination of hormones, and clinical trials have been looking at which formulation shuts off sperm production with the least side effects. One promising method is a sustained-released testosterone capsule that is injected under the skin. In clinical trials at the University of Washington, the capsule, which gradually releases hormones over a period of several months, has been shown to completely shut off the production of sperm—temporarily, that is—with only minimal side effects, like light weight gain. But more research is needed.

So, once a hormone-based male contraceptive pill or implant is commercially available, how many men will actually take it? One team of researchers sought to answer that question in 2005 by surveying more than nine thousand men in eight different countries. Overall, about 55 percent of respondents said they would be interested in taking some form of hormone-based birth control.

In the meantime, the medical community has some concerns. One is that men who end up using some form of hormonal birth control will be less likely to use condoms, increasing the odds that they or their partners might contract an STD. There is also some concern that the 45 percent of men who say they will not use hormonal birth control might lie to their partners and say they are using it, simply to persuade their partners to have unprotected sex—operating under the rationale that if the woman gets pregnant, it's still *her* problem.

Those potential problems eventually will have to be addressed.

In any case, the thought of a male birth-control pill brings to mind that old question that's often asked, jokingly, when traditional gender roles in a male-female relationship are perceived as being reversed: Who wears the pants in that relationship?

Perhaps one day that old, tired question will be tweaked to reflect a new reality: Who takes the pill in that relationship?

DO WOMEN'S MENSTRUAL CYCLES SYNCHRONIZE?

Mother Nature is sometimes all too eager to keep individuals in certain species of animals in harmony with one another.

Southeast Asian fireflies are known to gather in droves in mangrove trees and flash in unison, to the point where an entire tree will light up and then go dark in three-second cycles. Blue whales, Earth's largest mammals, synchronize the frequency of their sonic songs across vast oceanic distances. Male fiddler crabs court females by gathering around them and waving their claws in unison. And on a more cosmic level, the moon synchronizes its orbit around Earth, Venus returns to almost its exact spot between the sun and the Earth every eight years, and even distant stars light-years away can be seen wobbling in synchrony with their orbiting planets.

But perhaps the most puzzling instance of behavioral unity in nature may be menstrual synchrony, the idea that women who live together, ovulate together.

The notion dates at least back to 1971, when Dr. Martha K. McClintock, an experimental psychologist, published a study showing that the menstrual cycles of 135 women living in an all-female college dormitory tended to synchronize over time. McClintock and other scientists suggested it might have something to do with pheromones, chemicals that send messages by smell.

But almost immediately, the findings came under assault. Many critics argued that synchrony simply could not be possible when women often have cycles of different lengths. Over time, they pointed out, if one woman with a cycle of twenty-eight days is living with a woman who has a cycle of thirty days, then their cycles will naturally *appear* to converge as certain months go by—say, from January to June. It's very easy to see how the onset of the women's cycles can converge simply as a result of the changing number of days from one month to the next and, conversely, how they would subsequently diverge.

One study in the journal *Human Nature* looked at 186 women living in dorms for a full year and found no evidence for synchrony. The authors also reviewed the original 1971 study and argued that its findings were due to chance, a claim that other teams have echoed as well.

But the chorus of critics has been pushed back by a series of pro-synchrony studies and experiments that have added weight to McClintock's original findings. The phenomenon has been studied outside of dorms and living situations and shown to occur in offices. One study in 1999, for example, looked at fifty-one pairs of women who worked together in tight quarters and had minimal contact with other people during the day. After about one year, there was evidence that the cycles of the women in each pair tended to occur on average within 3.5 to 4.3 days of each other, while the onsets of coworkers who had less contact ranged more broadly, between 7.7 and 9.0 days of each other. "This is the first unequivocal demonstration of menstrual synchrony outside of the household," the authors proclaimed.

But perhaps the most striking line of support came when a team at the University of Chicago—which included McClintock—published a study in the journal *Nature* showing that compounds taken from the underarm secretions of healthy women who were in the early phases of their cycles could shorten the cycle of women exposed to the substances. When extracts were taken from the women while they were in midcycle, they had the opposite effect, effectively lengthening the menstrual cycles of other women. The effects were quick and drastic: in the first case, 68 percent of the women experienced shortened cycles (many of which shrank significantly), while in the second phase of the study, a different 68 percent of the women experienced extended cycles.

The experiments provided hard evidence not only for synchrony, but also for the existence of pheromones, a crucial piece of the puzzle. And there is more reason to believe that women can indeed be led by their noses. Swiss scientists discovered that women could sniff out genetic differences in potential mates.

When women were asked to smell T-shirts that different men had worn, they often ranked more favorably the shirts that belonged to men with dissimilar genes for major histocompatibility complex, a group of proteins involved in immunity to disease. The odors a woman preferred also tended to remind her of past and current partners.

Put aside the awful images of sniffing smelly T-shirts for a moment, and look at it from a scientific standpoint. Seeking out different immune-system genes might be a way to prevent inbreeding or to arm offspring with a more versatile immune system. Rachel S. Herz, a psychologist at Brown University, found that women ranked body odor above almost every other factor in attraction except "pleasantness." "For women, the costs of pregnancy, like time and energy, are pretty high," she explained to me. "So to balance those costs, you want to make sure the child is going to live. And what is indicative of how healthy you are is your immune system, which is manifested in your smell."

These patterns of sniff-and-mating are found not just in humans, but other animals as well, from moths and butterflies to mice and boars and, possibly, some primates. But if you accept that menstrual cycles in women can synchronize, as many scientists are now wont to, then a major question still remains: What's the purpose of it?

No one can say for sure. In laboratory experiments, scientists have found that menstrual synchrony benefits rats because they subsequently conceive, deliver, and raise their pups in groups. That allows the mothers to share rearing responsibilities, including lactation, which in turn benefits the offspring because they are nursed more often, allowing them to grow more quickly. Evolutionary scientists believe that while this wouldn't necessarily apply to women today, it certainly would have benefited mothers in ancient times.

CAN BICYCLE SEATS CAUSE IMPOTENCE IN WOMEN?

A Boston urologist sent shock waves through the cycling world when he declared in 1997 that there are two kinds of cyclists—"those who are impotent, and those who will be impotent."

It was not too long before a raft of studies showing a strong cause-and-effect relationship between bike seats and impotence emerged. As one friend who quickly but begrudgingly cut back on cycling told me, if you continued riding day in and day out, you'd soon be pedaling all the way to Flaccid City. Population: You.

But amid all the hubbub, there was one concern that seemed to go unaddressed. The studies that started the frenzy looked almost exclusively at male riders, and the warnings that grew out of their findings were all directed at men. Somehow, for some reason, women cyclists were left out of the mix.

Instead of being studied directly, it was simply assumed that women riders would suffer the same fate as their male counterparts. In men, traditional bike seats compress an artery and nerve that supply the genitals with blood and sensation. Like a flattened drinking straw, the nerve and artery lose their circular shape after being squashed one too many times, clearing the way for impotence to set in. Since women have the same nerve and artery—which, for them, play a role in engorging the clitoris during sex—many scientists believed women would also face higher rates of impotence after spending too much time in the bike saddle.

Then a study in 2006 showed, surprisingly, that that may not be the case at all. Led by an assistant professor at Yale medical school, the study team found that bike seats appear to affect women differently than men. Included in the research were forty-eight healthy, premenopausal cyclists who biked three to four days a week for about two hours, and had been cycling for an average of eight years. They were compared with twenty-two similarly healthy women whose recreational sport was jogging; they ran an average of five days a week for a distance of about four and a half miles.

Like male riders, many of the female riders in the study experienced tingling, pain, and decreased genital sensation. But they did not show symptoms of impaired sexual function. One possibility is that any serious sexual side effects might only become apparent in longer-term studies. But the findings may also reflect a lower susceptibility to sexual side effects among women than men, a result, for example, of anatomical differences that produce less compression when women are in the saddle. Or the nerve and artery that are compressed during riding and that are so important to sexual function in men may not be quite as critical to arousal in women.

In one sense, it is easy to see why. When it comes to sexuality, men and women are differently tuned. Consider that for almost a decade, researchers at Pfizer endeavored to show that Viagra, the male impotence drug, could enhance sexual function in women. Doing so would have allowed Pfizer to expand—perhaps even double—its base of customers for the little blue pill.

But in early 2004, they gave up.

Countless tests showed that for men, sexual arousal and desire are often intertwined. In men, increasing blood flow to the genitals, which is the task Viagra performs, is enough to spark desire—and, of course, vice versa. For women, however, the two are frequently distinct. Studies have shown that exposing women to sexual images can spark blood flow to the genitals, but it does not automatically lead to a conscious desire for sex. In one study at Northwestern University, women who were being exposed to sexual images reported feeling no sexual arousal at all, even though strategically placed devices said otherwise. What this proved is that in women, arousal and desire move largely in a single direction, on a one-way street: often, it is the mind that sets off physiological arousal. The reverse is not quite as successful.

That may help shed some light on the finding that women, unlike men, can experience decreased genital sensation without suffering impaired sexual function. Men and women are born not only with different machinery, but with different software instructions for running it. This may not come as a surprise to any long-married couple.

Can a woman be allergic to semen?

Unless you suffered from one of them yourself, you probably wouldn't believe some of the strange allergies that have been documented in the medical literature.

Just a few of the ones I've come across over the years are allergies to chocolate, beer, deodorant, frog meat, toothpaste, rabbits, and chamomile tea. In this age of wireless technology, one of the latest to emerge is an allergy to cell phones, which occurs when the nickel plating in some phones causes symptoms of contact dermatitis—like itchy rashes—on a person's ears and cheeks. This can also occur with MP3 players, which contain nickel as well.

But nothing quite takes the cake like seminal plasma protein hypersensitivity. Or in layman's terms, semen allergy. Odd as it may sound, there are plenty of women who discover that they're allergic to their sexual partner's semen. It occurs when antibodies in the woman's system respond negatively to certain proteins in the man's semen and attack them. These, I'm assuming, are the proteins that always leave the seat up, never listen, and constantly leave toenail clippings around the house.

As one medical report stated, "Allergic reactions to human seminal plasma protein have become increasingly recognized in the medical community."

Unfortunately, many women don't immediately realize that they have this allergy. Often it gets misdiagnosed as a recurrent yeast infection or even an STD, with symptoms like vaginal swelling, redness, itching, hives, blisters, or, in some cases, difficulty breathing. But one way a woman can tell is by using a condom a few times. If the symptoms always seem to coincide with sex, but go away when a condom is used, that's usually a pretty good sign of an allergy.

You can imagine that this would cause a lot of problems between a man and a woman who are trying to conceive. But it can and has been overcome. In mild cases, doctors can help desensitize a woman to her partner's semen through repeated exposure, sometimes using injections that are similar to conventional allergy shots. In more severe cases, women have been able to get pregnant through in vitro fertilization. It's expensive, but you can't really put a price tag on love, can you?

CAN HOT TUBS CAUSE INFERTILITY?

For years, doctors have warned men having trouble conceiving to stay away from hot baths and whirlpool tubs, saying there was reason to suspect that long exposure to hot water could worsen their problems.

Much of that was based on speculation. But in 2007, a team of urologists at the University of California at San Francisco conducted a study to measure and document the extent, if any, of this effect. The researchers did confirm the link, and then they discovered something surprising.

The study looked at a group of men who were regularly exposed to high water temperatures, roughly for about thirty minutes a week through hot tubs or hot baths. All the men showed signs of infertility, with impaired sperm production and motility.

What was unexpected was how quickly this infertility could be reversed. The researchers found that after the men stopped their exposure to wet heat, half had "a mean increase in total motile sperm counts of 491 percent after three to six months." Yes, 491 percent.

Among the men who did not see such a reversal, the researchers speculated that tobacco use, a known "gonadotoxic" habit, was to blame. Most of those men were regular smokers. As for women, there's no solid evidence that hot tubs can affect egg production or cause infertility. One might imagine that the female reproductive system might be slightly less susceptible than its male counterpart, since it doesn't exactly *hang* out there like a man's. But no one can say for certain. And there are some worrisome signs. One study in 2003 found that women who used hot tubs or Jacuzzis in early pregnancy were twice as likely to miscarry as women who did not.

The best advice: whether you're a man or a woman, if you're having trouble conceiving, try staying away from hot tubs for a little while.

DO KEGEL EXERCISES WORK?

They are known by many names, some more amusing than others: pelvic-floor presses, sexual squeezes, crotch crunches, and my personal favorite, crunches down under.

Call them what you want. But in the medical literature, at least, the act of repeatedly contracting and relaxing the muscles of the pelvic floor in order to strengthen them is known as a Kegel exercise, named after Dr. Arnold Kegel, the doctor who introduced it in 1948 as a way for women to control incontinence after childbirth. I can only assume Dr. Kegel had no idea the exercise would one day be widely used not simply among women looking to combat incontinence, but among those hoping to—let's see how I can put this delicately—enhance sexual gratification.

The best part about the exercise, so I'm told, is that it can be done anytime, anywhere, with no one knowing: in the office, at the desk, on the subway, in between courses at a restaurant, on a boring transatlantic flight. And you don't have to look too far or spend much time in many online sexual-health forums to find plenty of women who claim to do just that. As a female friend told me in conversation, "Lots of women claim they do them while they're talking to you, working, making a presentation, blah, blah, blah."

But like most women—and likely a lot of men, as well—my friend wanted to know: Do Kegels actually work? The short answer, it seems, is yes.

While there aren't many randomized, carefully controlled studies investigating whether men and women find more sexual satisfaction after researchers assign one group of women to do Kegels and others to abstain—perhaps because such a study would end up not in a medical journal, but an adult-rated magazine—there is evidence from related studies that Kegel exercises do have an effect. Most of the research is on women who suffer complications after a particularly difficult childbirth, such as incontinence or conditions like uterine and vaginal prolapse, which involve decreased muscle strength in the pelvic floor.

Most of the studies, including a large meta-analysis published in the *Cochrane Database of Systematic Reviews* in 2006 and a study of seventy-five women in 2005, have found that regularly engaging in pelvic-floor exercises like Kegels can reduce the severity of prolapse and build up muscle tone. Firming up these muscles means improved sex because it can result in a more intense orgasm, as well as a stronger grip (which benefits her partner).

So effective are Kegels, it seems, that urologists also recommend them for men who suffer from sexual dysfunction.

"These exercises, although primarily used for controlling

urinary incontinence," wrote two medical researchers at Tulane and Louisiana State University in a report in 2005, "have recently been found to be beneficial in treating premature ejaculation. These exercises are easy to perform and lack side effects, thus making it a widely acceptable therapeutic option. And unlike any drug therapy, the benefits are long term." And the muscles strengthened by Kegels also help control the firmness of a man's erection.

The researchers, Dr. Neil Baum and Bradley Spieler, offered the following technique for those, both men or women, looking for some pelvic strengthening:

1. To isolate the muscles, go to the bathroom and try to stop the flow of urine midstream. Do this several times so that you know what these muscles feel like.
2. To begin the exercises, you must have an empty bladder. Tightly contract the muscles you have just identified and hold them tight for ten seconds. Then relax the muscles for ten seconds.
3. Repeat this procedure ten times, approximately three times a day. It is important to identify correctly the involved muscle group; otherwise these exercises will not be useful.

ARE TWO CONDOMS BETTER PROTECTION THAN ONE?

Wearing two sweaters at the same time keeps you warmer in the winter than one, and doubling up on a pair of socks keeps your toes better protected against frostbite than a single pair. As the old saying goes, two is better than one.

But when it comes to condoms, it doesn't work that way. In fact, it may work in the reverse. Using two condoms can end up providing *less* protection, not more, because the friction between the two condoms during sex makes them each more likely to break or slip off. That applies to using two male condoms simultaneously or a male and a female condom at once.

Besides, while they may not look all that sturdy, individual condoms are in fact remarkably good at preventing unwanted pregnancies and STDs. According to Planned Parenthood, every year only two out of every one hundred women whose partners correctly use condoms become pregnant. When condoms are used incorrectly, however, the rate of women who become pregnant shoots way up, to about fifteen out of one hundred.

As for STDs, researchers at the National Institutes of Health report that correctly and consistently using condoms reduces the risk of contracting HIV by about 85 percent, and significantly reduces the risk of contracting other diseases as well.

For a thin piece of latex that you can get almost anywhere for free, that's pretty reliable.

So what happens if you do double up?

It's not clear precisely to what extent you'll affect the aforementioned odds, but the relevant statistics paint a grim picture. One study that looked at sexually active teenage girls in Kentucky found that errors or problems with condom usage "were significantly higher among teens diagnosed with a sexually transmitted disease." Another study by scientists at the Centers for Disease Control and Prevention looked at nearly 250 HIV-positive gay and bisexual men and found that about 35 percent had engaged in the practice of wearing two condoms.

So it seems that two is not always better than one after all. In this case, at least, one is exactly enough.

CAN A WOMAN GET PREGNANT DURING HER PERIOD?

I remember watching a television show not long ago about a woman who was trying to determine the father of her two children, a set of fraternal twins we'll call Jack and Elizabeth. The woman was sure it was one of two men, both of whom had reluctantly agreed to take paternity tests and appear on the show to hear the results. When the host opened the envelope and started reading the results—"John, in the case of two-year-old Elizabeth, you *are* the father"—the second man, Robert, jumped out of his chair and screamed in celebration, apparently relieved he was off the hook.

Not so fast. Two seconds later, the host went on: "Robert, in the case of two-year-old Jack, *you* are the father."

What? How could two different men be the fathers of one set of fraternal twins delivered by a single woman?

It turns out that as with all fraternal twins, Jack and Elizabeth came from two different eggs that their mother released at the same time (identical twins result from one fertilized egg splitting in half). But the mother had apparently had intercourse with two different men in a window of time that was narrow enough to allow each egg to be fertilized by a different man's sperm. Each fertilized egg, or zygote, then developed and matured, eventually resulting in the mother giving birth to fraternal twins who were half siblings!

Bizarre, isn't it?

I bring this up to illustrate the fact that the laws of human reproduction—or all reproduction, for that matter—can be strange and counterintuitive. What sounds unlikely, or just downright impossible, can sometimes very certainly occur. And that brings us to whether a woman can get pregnant during her period. It would seem on its face to be impossible, but it's not. While it is unlikely, some women can indeed get pregnant during their periods.

One reason is that women can sometimes have spotting during ovulation. So a woman may think she is having her period when she really isn't. Another reason is that some women have extremely short cycles. This causes them to ovulate, or release an egg, almost immediately after their period has finished, and some women may even ovulate before their menstrual bleeding has stopped. If a woman has unprotected sex during her period and an egg is present, it can be fertilized and result in pregnancy.

Or something else even more surprising can happen. Most people don't realize that sperm can survive in the female body for several days and, some experts say, as long as five days. They are extremely sturdy, versatile, determined—and plentiful. Hundreds of millions are typically released during a single ejaculation (as a friend once said, maybe it takes that many sperm to fertilize one egg because not one of the little guys will stop and ask for directions). If a woman has unprotected sex during her period and releases an egg shortly afterward, any lingering sperm could conceivably reach it.

In fact, according to a study of more than two hundred women by researchers at the National Institutes of Health, women not only can become pregnant during menstruation, but can get pregnant at virtually any time during their cycle. In the study, the scientists found that a woman can become fertile as early as the fourth day of her cycle, and that about a fifth of all women are fertile by the seventh day. It used to be thought that women were generally fertile between days ten and seventeen of their cycle.

Who knows what other assumptions we hold about sex and reproduction may also soon fall . . .

DOES CIRCUMCISION REDUCE SEXUAL PLEASURE?

Talk about a sensitive subject!

Just the mere mention of it is enough to provoke heated debate. Men who've had the procedure performed on them claim it's healthy and hygienic, pointing to research showing that it lowers the rate of urinary tract infections and STDs and has no effect on pleasure. Those who escaped the maternity ward with their foreskin intact say that the benefits of circumcision are overstated and ask how it'd be possible to lose foreskin that contains thousands of nerve endings *without* affecting sexual enjoyment. Then there are women, some who say they prefer the natural turtleneck and those who say they can do without it.

Fortunately, scientists have spent years doing research on this matter. Unfortunately, there is still no clear answer.

Most studies have tended to focus on populations of men who chose to undergo the procedure as adults for cosmetic, religious, or medical reasons, the thinking behind this being that they'd be able to describe any before-and-after changes (as opposed to someone who had the procedure, say, at three days old). Most of these men report decreased sensation, but surprisingly, some report this as a benefit—leading, for example, to longer and more enjoyable sex—while others call it a drawback.

In a study published in the journal *Urology* in 2002, scientists looked at 123 adult men who underwent the operation and found that most experienced both decreased sensitivity and improved satisfaction. "Over all," the report found, "62 percent were satisfied with having been circumcised." Three years later, a study of 150 men carried out by British urologists found that 38 percent of newly circumcised men experienced improved sensation after circumcision, while 18 percent reported less sensation and another 44 percent experienced no change.

But for every study suggesting reduced sexual pleasure, another argues the opposite. Take, for example, one that was published in 2008, which included thousands of men: "Adult male circumcision was not associated with sexual dysfunction. Circumcised men reported increased penile sensitivity and enhanced ease of reaching orgasm."

One theory is that the important variable here, "pleasure," is something that varies tremendously from one man to the next. And since circumcision, the procedure itself, is something of an inexact science, the results for each circumcised man will differ.

Suffice it to say that the research is so conflicting that it's impossible to draw any decisive conclusion. The American Academy of Family Physicians, which issued a report on circumcision in 2007, may have said it best.

"The effect of circumcision on penile sensation or sexual satisfaction is unknown. Because the epithelium of a circumcised glans becomes cornified, and because some feel nerve over-stimulation leads to desensitization, many believe that the glans of a circumcised penis is less sensitive," the authors write. But, they go on, "No valid evidence to date, however, supports the notion that being circumcised affects sexual sensation or satisfaction."

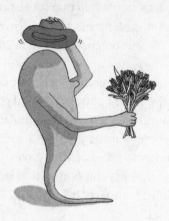

6
SPERM MEETS EGG
And Other Baby Matters

There are three times in life when you are virtually guaranteed to receive unsolicited advice—advice that's not only unsolicited but perhaps even strange or unhelpful, if not both.

One, I have learned, is any time you step onto a golf course as a novice. I can count on one hand the number of times in my life I have attempted to play golf, and yet I have lost count of the number of exchanges I've had on the green that began with, "Hey, you know you're holding that putter wrong. Move your hand up on it. . . . No, not like that. Okay, just hand the thing over and I'll show you!" This, I believe, is how golfers secretly keep all those outsiders from invading their clubs.

The second is the period between an engagement and a wedding. When it comes to planning a wedding, everyone seems to know what will work best for *your* wedding—whether it's the flower arrangement, the music, the location, the food, or the centerpieces. And if it's the bride or groom's parents who are covering the costs, well, you've got no choice but to listen, and occasionally acquiesce.

The third occasion, it seems, is during pregnancy.

I know what you're thinking. First, off, I'm a dude. And second, what could I possibly know about pregnancy, considering that, at least at the time of this writing, I don't have any children. But I'm also a health reporter, and writing a column that explores old wives' tales and all sorts of health-related peculiarities puts me in a unique position. There seem to be an awful lot of old wives' tales about making babies.

And despite the fact that we now know a great deal about exactly how pregnancies occur, these issues seem to end up near the top of the list of people's nagging health questions.

Many of those questions begin with, "My friends told me," "The other day my mother insisted," and the ever popular, "I am constantly being told by strangers that . . ."

It seems that everyone has some bit of pregnancy-related folklore or wisdom stored up, and they insist on sharing it when the opportunity arises. They include the outlandish, like the one that says you're having a boy if your legs are as thick as tree trunks and a girl if they're firm and fit. Or the one that says that you're having a girl if you're crabby because women tend to be crabbier and having a girl inside you only multiplies the crabbiness. (Hey, I don't come up with them—I just repeat 'em!) Others are not quite as absurd, but still leave you scratching your head, wondering why—and how—they could be true, like the one about morning sickness being a sign of a healthy pregnancy, or the way you're carrying your pregnancy predicting the sex of your baby.

And why shouldn't we be intensely interested? Most members of the animal kingdom spend their entire lives pursuing reproductive success, with some even sacrificing their lives for little more than a mere *shot* at mating. Male praying mantises will often approach females with caution, as female mantises are sometimes known to bite off and consume the male's head after copulation. Scorpions and spiders have been observed engaging in similar acts. And Pacific salmon, those delicious swimming sushi rolls to be, leap and struggle to make their way upstream to spawn, only to die shortly after laying their eggs as a result of all the exhaustion and stress they incurred during their gallant journey.

There are scientists who feel strongly that many of us humans, too, carry a similar posterity-at-all-costs streak somewhere in the subconscious as well. We may not sacrifice our lives for a mere shot at reproducing, but many parents would put their children first at all costs. We just care about our lineage that much, it seems.

That may be why pregnancy inspires such intense curiosity, even between strangers. Or perhaps we just like to play the gender guessing game. Either way, the next time you or your partner gets pregnant, you're bound to be besieged with all sorts of strange, amusing, and perhaps even fascinating bromides. You may as well go into it prepared.

DOES MOTHER'S HEARTBURN MEAN A HAIRY NEWBORN?

It's an odd adage that has stuck around longer than anyone can remember. If an expectant mother suffers heartburn so badly that it feels like she swallowed a jalapeno, there's a good chance she'll have a baby with a head that's hairy enough to cause rug burn. But doctors have long shrugged it off as just another case of pregnancy folklore.

Until now, that is. After decades of telling expectant mothers not to buy into the saying, researchers at Johns Hopkins University conducted a study intending to finally, once and for all, put the claim to rest. To their surprise, they ended up confirming it.

The study, published in the journal *Birth* in 2006, followed sixty-four pregnant women, about 78 percent of whom reported having some heartburn. After the women gave birth, two outside observers looked at pictures of their infants and rated their levels of hair.

Of the twenty-eight women who reported moderate to severe heartburn, twenty-three had newborn babies with average or above-average amounts of hair. Conversely, ten of the twelve women who reported no heartburn had babies with little or no hair. Obviously the results showed that this is by no means a hard-and-fast rule. About 82 percent of the women who had moderate to severe heartburn birthed hairy babies, while 18 percent did not. But it's enough to suggest there's a strong relationship between heartburn and hairy babies.

The obvious question is, why?

The reason appears to be that in pregnant women, high levels of estrogen and other hormones can relax the sphincter at the bottom of the esophagus, which triggers heartburn. Many of these same hormones have been shown to influence the rate of fetal hair growth. Which means that more of these hormones can mean more fetal hair, and in turn, more heartburn. "Contrary to expectations, it appears that an association between heartburn severity during pregnancy and newborn hair does exist," the researchers wrote. "We propose a shared biologic mechanism involving a dual role of pregnancy hormones in both the relaxation of the lower esophageal sphincter and the modulation of fetal hair growth."

In a conversation, Kathleen Costigan, a registered nurse who runs the fetal assessment center at Johns Hopkins and was the study's lead author, said expectant mothers had been trying for years to convince her that there was a connection. But she always dismissed it, she said, and encouraged her patients not to listen to the numerous myths about pregnancy floating around. She had hoped that her study would provide the hard evidence she could point to when her pregnant patients came to her office looking for extrastrength antacids and advice on where to buy a pair of baby-safe hair clippers.

So the findings, you might imagine, came as a shock. "We've heard this claim hundreds of times, and I've always told people that it's nonsense," she told me. "Since the study came out, I've had to eat a lot of crow."

CAN SEXUAL POSITION DURING CONCEPTION DETERMINE A BABY'S SEX?

When it comes to sex, there is generally one position that most people can believe in: yes, please! When it comes to sex for couples who are trying to conceive and looking for a way to get a child of a particular gender, there's an entirely different story. True, they could always turn to a sympathetic fertility clinic. But couples who want a lower-tech method have often been told they can succeed in their quest with a calendar and the right position.

Much of the talk is tied to a technique called the Shettles method, popularized in the 1970s, which holds that couples can indeed increase their odds of having the gender they prefer by choosing the right timing and position. The premise is that sperm carrying the X and Y chromosomes have different characteristics, and that each is likely to fertilize the egg—which is always X— under different circumstances. Male sperm, which carry the small Y chromosome, are supposedly fast and fragile, while female sperm, carrying the much bigger X chromosome, are slow swimmers but nonetheless sturdier. As a result, the theory holds, if you want to have a boy, you should have sex as close to ovulation as possible and in a position that leads to deeper penetration. To have a girl, on the other hand, have sex two to three days before ovulation, and choose a position that creates shallow penetration, preferably the missionary position.

The reasoning? Shallow penetration means sperm are deposited closer to the vaginal entrance, where the environment is acidic and the strong, female sperm have a better chance of survival. Deeper penetration, on the other hand, favors the quick male sperm because it deposits them closer to the egg—away from the harsh environment at the entrance, enabling them to step on the gas and reach the egg first. Supporters of this method, and similar ones, claim a success rate as high as 90 percent.

But don't count on it. Several studies have tried to confirm the claim and found no effect. In 1991, researchers, again at Johns Hopkins University, analyzed the findings of six previous studies on the subject. They found that relying on timing and position for "natural family planning" didn't work.

A later study, in the *New England Journal of Medicine*, followed 221 healthy women who were planning a pregnancy. Of those, 192 became pregnant during the study period. Again, the researchers found no timing effect. "There were no systematic differences between the patterns of intercourse that produced boys and the patterns that produced girls," the authors wrote.

On the bright side, whether it's a boy or a girl you specifically want, you'll always have good odds. There's a 50 percent chance you'll get what you want. But then again, every baby—regardless of sex—is a precious gift, something most new parents discover before the cord is even cut.

CAN YOU PREDICT THE SEX OF A BABY BY THE WAY THE MOTHER IS CARRYING?

If the woman's carrying low, it's a boy. If she's carrying high, it's a girl. If she's carrying all the weight out front in the shape of a basketball, it's a boy. If the shape of her belly is strangely reminiscent of a watermelon, then it's probably a girl.

These are not exactly scientific assertions, but they've persisted for so long, over so many centuries, that they're widely accepted fact. (Well, except for the comparison to a basketball, which is the modern interpretation.) Some parents-to-be are so convinced of the logic behind these predictions that they paint a baby's room pink or blue—depending on the shape and height of the belly—before the sex has even been categorically determined by amniocentesis, ultrasound, or delivery.

So where does this come from? According to Dr. Jonathan Schaffir, an assistant professor of obstetrics and gynecology at Ohio State University who studies pregnancy-related old wives' tales, the claim has its origins in Hippocrates' days, when it was believed that male fetuses were conceived on the right and girls on the left. How Hippocrates conceived this one is not entirely clear, but as the so-called Father of Medicine, it's safe to say his judgment was rarely questioned. He was the first to identify the symptoms of a number of chronic diseases and is the first documented chest surgeon, and even today, centuries later, many of the treatments and procedures he introduced are still widely used.

Besides, on its face at least, the notion that how the mother carries might say something about the sex of the baby sounds more reasonable than some of the other gender-prediction claims floating around, among them that a mother can tell the sex by the type of food she craves, spicy for boys and sweet for girls.

Revered as the method may be, it has no real scientific footing. In one large 1999 study, for example, researchers at Johns Hopkins recruited 104 pregnant women who did not know the sex of their babies and put the maxim to the test: they found that the shape of the abdomen was a poor predictor of a baby's sex. It worked roughly 50 percent of the time—the equivalent of a random guess.

But some findings were unexpected. Women with more than twelve years of education correctly predicted the sex of their babies about 70 percent of the time, compared with 43 percent of the time for less educated women. And hunches that were based on dreams and feelings, it turned out, were more accurate than those based on the way a woman carried. But the authors had no idea why.

So why do some women carry high and others carry low? The shape and height of the belly is determined not by sex, but by muscle tone and the baby's position. And when a woman is carrying low, it often means quite simply that the mother is nearing delivery and the baby is inching closer to the birth canal. It's a sign that a trip to the paint store will soon be required, but it won't tell you whether you should buy pink or blue.

IS MORNING SICKNESS A SIGN OF A HEALTHY PREGNANCY? DOES IT MEAN A GREATER LIKELIHOOD OF HAVING A GIRL?

It may be among the most dreaded aspects of pregnancy, but perhaps many women would look differently at morning sickness if they knew it was an indication of a lower risk of miscarriage, a not so pleasant sign, as it were, that both mother and unborn child were protected. Or that it might tip them off to the baby's gender.

Indeed, that may very well be the case. A widespread belief going back decades holds that morning sickness, a condition that affects two-thirds of women worldwide, can be a sort of blessing in disguise, or at least a favorable omen. While many tales about pregnancy have been crushed by the weight of contradictory scientific evidence, these two, it seems, appear to be exceptions.

Pregnant women who find themselves crouched at the toilet morning in and morning out might find at least a sliver of solace in the fact that studies have shown that they may be less likely to miscarry. One prominent study, published in 2007, followed nearly seven thousand pregnant women and discovered that those who had nausea in their first trimesters were an eye-popping 70 percent less likely to miscarry. That supported the findings of a study published a year earlier that found that women who had morning sickness had a significantly lower risk of miscarriage, but not low birth weight, preterm delivery, and other adverse outcomes.

So why would something so awful be associated with something so wonderful?

No one can say for sure. But it has been shown that increased nausea and vomiting are linked to higher levels of a hormone produced by healthy placental tissue, and a prevailing theory suggests that the sickness may be an evolutionary survival mechanism with converse side effects, much like the gene for sickle cell anemia, which has the surprising upside of protecting against malaria. In this case it seems that nausea and vomiting may help pregnant women avoid foods that are harmful to developing fetuses—a particularly crucial measure of protection when you consider that pregnant women's immune systems are weaker during their first trimesters so the odds of the fetal tissue being rejected as foreign are lowered.

Some scientists have gone so far as to say that morning sickness is no sickness at all, but security. One exhaustive study by researchers at Cornell University found that pregnant women have the greatest aversions to foods most likely to harbor infectious and toxic organisms—specifically meats, fish, poultry, and eggs. Many women also have aversions to alcoholic and caffeinated beverages, like coffee, which have all been linked to a heightened risk of miscarriage, and studies show that women who vomit experience fewer miscarriages than those who suffer solely from nausea.

If that weren't intriguing enough, there's more. The Cornell scientists sifted through sixty years of data to show that, compared to industrial societies where morning sickness is prevalent, nonindustrial societies with nonexistent or exceptionally low rates of the condition are significantly less likely to have meat as a dietary staple and much more likely, instead, to have corn as a staple. Consider, for example, that the industrialized nation with the highest rate of morning sickness—a country where roughly nine in ten pregnant women reportedly experience the condition—is Japan. Is there any nation with a greater affinity for consuming raw fish, a habit that increases the risk of exposure to fetal-threatening compounds like mercury, PCBs (polychlorinated biphenyl), and parasites?

To be sure, other scientists have proposed alternate theories for the cause of morning sickness. Some have argued that it is meant to warn potential sexual partners, as well as relatives who might offer assistance, that the woman is pregnant. And still others with a psychoanalytic bent have suggested it may be some sort of Freudian process by which an expectant mother expresses her frustration toward the unborn child and father who have saddled her with such pain and discomfort.

No doubt interesting. But unlike the notion of morning sickness protecting against pathogens, neither of these alternate theories is backed by any hard evidence.

As for morning sickness predicting a baby's gender, there's good reason to believe it's more fact than fantasy. A number of large studies in various countries have examined whether it can sometimes indicate that a girl is on the way, and almost all have found it to be true, albeit with a couple of caveats. Specifically, it seems only to apply to women whose morning sickness occurs in the first trimester, and with symptoms so severe that it leads to hospitalization, a condition known as hyperemesis gravidarum.

One of the largest studies was conducted by epidemiologists at the University of Washington. In it, the scientists compared 2,110 pregnant women who were hospitalized with morning sickness in their first trimesters to a control group of 9,783 women who did not get severely ill. They found that the women who got sick were more likely to deliver a girl, and that those who were the sickest—hospitalized for three days or more—had the greatest odds: a staggering increase of 80 percent compared to the control women. It's a finding that's been replicated many times.

But in this case there may not be any evolutionary advantages. More simply, it's known that female babies produce different hormones than male babies, and higher levels of these hormones—some of which are still being identified—cause slightly more illness than those that are elevated by male babies.

CAN FETAL HEART RATE PREDICT THE SEX OF THE BABY?

While the old wives who were spouting wisdom were clearly preoccupied with childbirth, nowadays medical literature is becoming just as rife with claims about unusual, new ways to predict the sex of an unborn baby.

One that has been around for decades, and has even gained some acceptance, is the idea that fetal heartbeat is faster among girls. Rates above 140 beats per minute are supposedly typical for girls; below that, look for a boy. With the emergence of technologies like fetal sonography and personal computers in the 1980s, expectant parents quickly took an interest in learning fetal heart rates and any other measurement that could tell them anything about their unborn babies.

But why faster heart rates for girls and slower beats for boys? I for one am inclined to believe it has its origins in gender stereotypes. Racked with excitement, adrenaline coursing through her veins and sending her tiny heart aflutter, the female baby cannot wait to get out and take on the world, like a tiny Mary Tyler Moore ready to explore. Male babies, however, are inclined to take it easy and relax (hey, what's the rush?) as they hang out Al Bundy–style on the gestational couch, as it were.

That's just my opinion. The exact source of the claim still remains a mystery. But what *has* become clear from various studies is that the belief holds little water.

Typically, the embryonic heart rate starts out at about 85 beats per minute and then accelerates at a rate of roughly three beats per minute each day during the first month. After the rate reaches an average of about 175 beats per minute, studies show, the acceleration reverses; by the middle of pregnancy, the rate averages 120 to 160 beats per minute.

That goes for both girls and boys. In one study published in the *British Journal of Obstetrics and Gynaecology*, researchers studied fetal heart-rate variations in seventy-nine women, looking for differences between male and female fetuses. They could not find any, but the search was not entirely fruitless. It was shown that during and after labor, the female heart rate increases considerably. Why, nobody knows. Curiously, scientists have also seen evidence that the fetal heartbeat can speed up in response to changes in a pregnant woman's blood pressure and levels of anxiety, as if there were some sort of emotional placenta capable of transmitting information about the mother's psychological state to the baby. That, or chronic anxiety, releases certain hormones that flow across the placenta and directly affect the baby.

Fetal heart rate may not tell us much about gender, but perhaps one day we will view it as a sort of barometer of a woman's psychological health. And those sudden kicks and turns that mothers often sense without warning may turn out to be messages from fetus to mother: calm down out there, you're making *me* anxious too.

DO IDENTICAL TWINS HAVE IDENTICAL DNA?

It is a basic tenet of human biology, taught in grade schools everywhere: identical twins come from the same fertilized egg, which splits neatly into two mirror-image halves, and thus, they share identical genetic profiles.

But it's time to rewrite the biology books. What you learned in school was wrong.

Though identical twins share very similar genes, identical they are not. It's a realization that only came about in recent years as scientists probed and compared the genomes of identical twins, wondering why two people who hail from the same embryo can differ in phenotype, as biologists refer to a person's physical manifestation. Consider, for example, that in some pairs, one identical twin may develop a disease with a genetic role or basis, while the other does not.

For a long time, most scientists explained away these discrepancies between identical twins as solely the result of environment, not any underlying genetic differences. Bolstering that argument was research that showed that some of these differences can spring from unique changes in what are known as epigenetic factors, the chemical markers that attach to genes and affect how they are expressed—in some cases acting as brake pads that slow or shut the genes off, and in others by acting as the accelerator that increases their output.

These epigenetic changes—which accumulate over a lifetime and can arise from things like diet and tobacco smoke—have been implicated in the development of cancer and behavioral traits like fearfulness and confidence, among other things. Epigenetic markers vary widely from one person to another, but identical twins were still considered genetically the same because epigenetics influence only the expression of a gene and not the underlying sequence of the gene itself. Simply put, they're the light fixtures on a house, not the frame.

But then it was revealed that epigenetic differences are only a part of the explanation. In 2008, scientists at the University of Alabama at Birmingham and at universities in Sweden and the Netherlands turned conventional wisdom on its ear with a stunning discovery. By examining the genes of ten pairs of identical twins, including nine pairs in which one twin showed signs of dementia or Parkinson's disease and the other did not, they showed that differences between identical twins run far deeper than the ornamental epigenetic markers: they occur way down at the very foundation. "When we started this study, people were expecting that only epigenetics would differ greatly between twins," Jan Dumanski, an author of the study, told me. "But what we found are changes on the genetic level, the DNA sequence itself."

At the core of these differences, the researchers found, is what geneticists call copy number variations, a phenomenon in which a gene exists in multiple copies, or a set of coding letters in DNA is missing. Not known, however, is whether these changes in identical twins occur mostly at the embryonic level, as the twins age, or both. But it's known that at least some of them begin immediately after conception.

After an egg is formed and fertilized, it must break apart into two separate cells in order to develop into two separate identical twins (fraternal twins, on the other hand, come from two different eggs that are fertilized at the same time). As the two halves of the egg develop into an embryo, they multiply constantly, producing more and more individual cells, each with its own copy of the organism's genome. But as the cells split repeatedly, they're prone to make mistakes in the number of copies of different genes that they pass on—much like someone divvying up a cake with a knife is bound to cut slices that are not entirely equal. One twin may make too many copies of gene A, while the second twin may replicate gene A perfectly but make too many copies of gene B, and so forth. The result is that a pair of identical twins will have extremely similar—but certainly not identical—sets of DNA. This distinction, along with environmental influences that occur over time, are the reasons that anyone who spends enough time around a set of identical twins can eventually spot small differences that distinguish them.

If these copy number variations sound fairly minor, they are not. Some copy variations have been shown in humans to confer protection against diseases like AIDS, while others are believed to contribute to autism, lupus, and other conditions. By studying pairs of identical twins in which one sibling has a disease and the other does not, scientists should be able to identify more easily the genes involved in a number of deadly diseases. "Copy number variations were discovered only a few years ago, but they are immensely important," Dr. Carl Bruder, another author of the study, explained.

John Witte, a professor of genetic epidemiology at the University of California at San Francisco, said the discovery that identical twins are not exactly identical is part of a growing focus on genetic changes after the parents' template has been laid. This and other research, Witte said, shows "you've got a little bit more genetic variation than previously thought."

In the meantime, those biology textbooks need updating.

Dumanski pointed out to me, for example, that even as his study was being printed and distributed in the *American Journal of Human Genetics*, the following statement could be found on the Web site of the National Human Genome Research Institute, the group that financed the government project to decode the human genome: "Most of any one person's DNA, some 99.9 percent, is exactly the same as any other person's DNA. (Identical twins are the exception, with 100 percent similarity)."

That, we now know, is not the case.

Do twins always skip a generation?

Now that we know that identical twins aren't exactly identical after all, a couple of other common perceptions about twins could use some clearing up as well. People with twins in their extended families, for example, may be wondering whether a crib for two is in their future too.

According to conventional wisdom, twins not only run in families, but they also—for some strange reason—always skip at least one generation. It's a claim that's widely repeated, but only partly true.

Scientists have known for some time that there is a gene that can predispose women to hyperovulation, the act of releasing two or more eggs in a single menstrual cycle. When both eggs are fertilized, the resulting siblings are fraternal twins. And because this gene can be passed on, the tendency to have fraternal twins can in fact run in families—but only on the maternal side, since men obviously don't ovulate (or shouldn't, at least).

Identical twins, on the other hand, result from one fertilized egg randomly splitting in two. Because there is no known gene that influences the act of the egg splitting, it's considered a mere coincidence when one extended family has multiple sets of identical twins.

So what about the notion that twins always skip a generation?

Also a myth. It's an illusion that most likely arose because men who inherit the hyperovulation gene from their mothers are unaffected by it, but can still pass it on to their daughters, who, in turn, will have an increased likelihood of conceiving twins.

As someone who has a brother *and* a sister who each have a set of identical twin daughters—all four of them beautiful, but handfuls—finding out that I still don't have an unusually high likelihood of fathering identical twins is something of a relief.

DOES A NEW MOTHER REALLY LOSE A TOOTH AND GAIN A CHILD?

Oh, the wonders of a new baby: the birth of a new life, a blossoming family, a doting mother and father. But then there are those things that it can take away: hours and hours of free time, precious sleep at night, and, according to an old wives' tale that may be as old as the word pregnancy itself, a tooth or two for Mom.

The age-old claim holds that for every baby a woman has, she is bound to lose a tooth because the pregnancy interferes with her ability to absorb calcium, which goes mostly instead to the fetus to help develop its bones and teeth.

That explanation may be a stretch. But studies have in fact found a strong link between pregnancy and dental problems. Pregnant women do in fact have a heightened rate of tooth loss, gingivitis, and cavities, but not for the reasons most people think.

Much of it has to do with the pregnancy-induced surge of hormones—estrogen and progesterone in particular—that increase blood flow to the gums and cause inflammation, making them swollen, more sensitive, and likely to bleed easily. This in turn can prompt the gum tissue to respond in exaggerated ways to plaque that is already on the teeth. According to the American Academy of Periodontology, these problems usually develop in the second and third months of pregnancy and get worse up through to labor.

One study that demonstrated this was carried out by researchers at the New York University College of Dentistry in 2005, and presented at the eighty-third general session of the International Association for Dental Research. The scientists looked at 2,635 pregnant women in the United States and found not only that most had dental problems, but also that as the number of children a woman had increased, so too did her odds of having periodontal disease, missing teeth, and untreated cavities.

A large part of the effect appears to be a direct result of the surge of hormones during pregnancy, but there are other factors as well. Unfounded fears about the hazards that radiographs and drug interactions can pose to the fetus keep many women away from the dentist's chair. A study in 2001 by scientists at the Centers for Disease Control and Prevention, for example, found that although roughly a quarter of pregnant women surveyed reported having dental problems, just half sought treatment.

The other part of the problem stems from those notorious pregnancy food cravings. Constant snacking on junk food and sugary beverages can cause a buildup of plaque and cavity-inducing bacteria. Mothers with several children are particularly vulnerable because they're more likely to partake of the junk food that their children are eating.

The solution? Pregnant women should be vigilant about keeping their teeth clean, which means brushing with fluoride toothpaste at least twice a day, but preferably after every meal, and scheduling appointments with the dentist once during the first trimester and again during the second trimester. Visit more often if need be. Besides, why not get to know the dentist who'll soon be treating your toddler?

IS A BABY'S FEVER JUST A SIGN OF TEETHING?

Children. God bless their hearts. Parents spend the first two years of their kids' lives eagerly encouraging them to walk and talk at every moment—and the next twenty years telling them to sit down and keep quiet.

But few things can make a parent feel more helpless in those first blissful months than knowing the baby is in pain and not knowing what to do about it. That, I can only imagine, is how the belief that a crying, feverish baby isn't always a cause for concern came about. Chalk it up to teething, pay little mind, and go back to sleep, the advice goes. Teething is unavoidable, necessary, and there's nothing you can do about it. So call it a night.

A little wishful thinking, perhaps.

Either way, it's bad advice. That's because what might seem

like simple teething-related fever can actually be a symptom of a more serious problem, like a viral illness. And while the emergence of new teeth in infants under one year old can sometimes cause a slight increase in body temperature, studies show it does not generally cause a high-grade fever.

In 2000, a Cleveland Clinic team published a study in *Pediatrics* that followed 125 children from their four-month doctors' visits to their first birthdays. In that time, 475 tooth eruptions occurred, and the study found many symptoms in the roughly eight-day periods in which the teeth emerged like increased biting, drooling, gum rubbing, rashes on the face, and decreased appetite. But no teething children had a high-grade fever, 104 degrees Fahrenheit (40 degrees Celsius) or above.

A later study in *Pediatrics* followed children six months to thirty months old, with the same conclusion. There was no link between teething and body temperature or high fever. "Before caregivers attribute any infants' signs or symptoms of a potentially serious illness to teething," the first study said, "other possible causes must be ruled out."

Will rubbing alcohol help cool a baby's fever?

Getting a baby checked out for what seems like a routine fever may add more work to the lives of already overburdened parents. But if a baby in pain can leave the parents feeling helpless, then knowing the child has been treated and soothed may allow for a more peaceful night of sleep—at least until the child starts up again. When that happens, many parents have been known to employ a little rubbing alcohol to save the day.

We've already seen, in my earlier book, *Never Shower in a Thunderstorm*, that another type of alcohol, whiskey, won't do the trick. But is rubbing alcohol any better?

Rubbing, or isopropyl, alcohol may sting when poured on cuts and scrapes, but its cooling effects on intact skin have lent it a reputation as a quick home remedy against fevers in small children. According to a recent report in the journal *Pediatrics*, the folk treatment seems especially common among parents in low-income and minority communities, where it is passed down through generations and in some cases recommended by doctors.

As rubbing alcohol evaporates from skin, it soothes like a fresh breeze, potentially reducing body temperature. Many parents soothe their feverish children by rubbing it on the skin or adding a little to a sponge bath.

But using it this way can cause serious harm. Isopropyl alcohol is quickly absorbed through the skin, and large amounts applied topically can be inhaled, which can lead to alcohol poisoning and other problems. A number of case reports in the medical literature describe small children who slipped into comas after a caregiver used rubbing alcohol to reduce their fevers. Other reports have described cases in which adults suffered cardiac and neurological problems after using alcohol-soaked towels to cool down or ease pain.

For better results, try plain and simple acetaminophen (aspirin, in rare cases, can cause Reye's syndrome in children, which can be fatal) and a lukewarm bath—sans the rubbing alcohol.

DO BABIES BLINK LESS THAN ADULTS?

Parents of newborn children sometimes notice an unusual phenomenon. Normal babies rarely close their eyes, except, of course, when sleeping.

Considering the world of visual stimuli to which infants are suddenly exposed, and the range of primitive reflexes they typically display—forcibly sucking on objects put in their mouths, grasping things put in their hands, and throwing out their arms when startled—frequent blinking may seem natural for an infant. But studies show that they blink spontaneously at a rate far below that of adults.

One study, published in the *Annals of Neurology*, measured spontaneous blinking in 269 children and 179 adults. The researchers found that infants blink on average less than twice a minute, a rate that steadily increases up to the age of fourteen or fifteen. Adults, on average, blink about ten to fifteen times a minute.

One theory is that infants, whose ability to see is incomplete, work hard to soak in visual information.

Blinking serves primarily to coat the eyes with tears and remove any dirt or debris from the surface of the cornea. So another theory is that infants, perhaps because their eyes are better protected by smaller openings or because they sleep so much, require less eye lubrication. Whatever the reason, it may explain why so many infants appear so wide-eyed and filled with wonder.

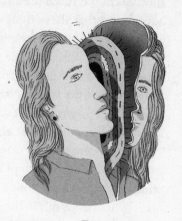

7

ATTACK OF THE BODY INVADERS

Following the Five-Second Rule

My eyes are open, but I am far from awake.

Clutching my head, I roll over and try to make sense of the grating noise that's broken the bedroom silence and roused me from a deep, peaceful sleep. Actually, it wasn't exactly deep, and it certainly wasn't peaceful. Rolling over, I launch an arm toward the night table and catch a glimpse of the time: 7:15 A.M. Time to go to work.

Minutes later, I'm on the train. Ordinarily the express shoots me from my home to Times Square so rapidly that I barely have time to be bothered by the fact that I'm being compressed into an object the size of a marble by the two thousand passengers who've squeezed into a subway car designed to hold no more than fifty people. But today it couldn't move fast enough. Nothing like having your face pressed into a cold, metal pole in the middle of a subway car. I'd reach for a handrail but I'm fairly certain studies have found that these things fall behind only public bathrooms and stripper poles when ranked by their level of cleanliness.

I begin to feel a sneeze coming on and struggle to stifle it. (Then I remember how harmful that can be—or so I've heard, repeatedly, over the years.) Not that it matters anymore, because a second later my reflexes overtake my self-control and *Thar She Blows!* As if my day hadn't already been off to a rough start.

The passenger who was subjected to this and appears to be from out of town—perhaps because of his I HEART NEW YORK hat, which no actual New Yorker in the history of New York has ever actually worn—is not in the least bit amused.

"Sorry man, total accident. But don't worry," I explain to him, "I don't have a cold or anything. It's just allergies."

I leave out the part about me being allergic to overcrowded subway cars. And it could very well be a cold. Not that I'd know either way, since it's often impossible to differentiate between allergies and a cold most of the time anyway, right? *That's something for me to look into when I finally make it to the newsroom.* I glance once again at my accidental victim, feeling even more sympathetic than I was a moment ago.

"Sorry buddy," I offer once more. *Still heart New York?*

SHOULD YOU FEED A COLD AND STARVE A FEVER?

Every year, when winter brings its dreary, mucky, frigid weather, an old maxim—one of the most quoted medical maxims around—is put to the test: feed a cold, starve a fever.

Wait: Or is it, starve a cold, feed a fever?

Actually, it may be neither. There are claims that the saying came to us by way of Hippocrates, and that its original form was,

"If you feed a cold, you will have to starve a fever." But that doesn't help make things any clearer.

There are two overriding schools of thought on the matter. One is that colds are a result of cold temperatures, and that in order to beat one you have to get your internal fire going by fueling the flames with food. By this same theory, a fever, since it arises or is associated with internal temperatures that are too high, must be snuffed out by starvation, much like a fire deprived of fuel or oxygen eventually dwindles. Then there are those who argue that the saying arises from the observation that a fever typically strips its victim of his or her appetite, while a cold does not.

Either way, many doctors and scientists have derided the saying over the years. But one good study, by a team of Dutch scientists and published in 2002 in the journal *Clinical and Diagnostic Laboratory Immunology*, has examined the issue. In it, the researchers found that eating a meal more than quadrupled the subjects' levels of gamma interferon, a protein molecule that our cells produce in response to viral infections, signaling that the immune system was shifting into high gear and more capable of fighting off a cold. But fasting, they discovered, prompted levels of gamma interferon to slide a bit while setting off a fourfold spike in levels of interleukin-4, which is exactly the response needed to fight off the bacterial infections that are typically the cause of most fevers. That suggests that gluttony during a fever might only prolong the suffering.

Others who are reluctant to alter their advice to patients have argued that the findings have little merit because the study involved a small number of subjects and has not been replicated. For now, most doctors say there is only one tried-and-true treatment: plenty of rest and fluids, and that goes for both cold *and* flu sufferers. Once a person has contracted either, the sickness will run its course in five to ten days.

Replication may be the cornerstone of good research, but I know there are those who will stick to the old maxim. For the holdouts, it may be wise, as a fellow New Yorker once exhorted, to follow the advice of turn-of-the-century physician Sir William Osler, considered one of the luminaries of modern medicine: "The cold should not be treated with contempt, but followed by bed rest, a good book to read, no food."

CAN A CUP OF TEA CLEAR UP YOUR CHEST?

What should you feed your cold, anyway? Like ice for a burn or a lozenge for a cough, a cup of hot tea is the age-old balm for sniffles, sneezing, and stuffiness.

Hot liquids, it is said, help loosen secretions in the chest and sinuses, making them easier to expel and ultimately clearing up congestion. The fluids are also meant to reverse dehydration. But only recently have scientists examined whether the effect is real. And boy, would Mama be proud.

Researchers at—where else!—the Common Cold Center at Cardiff University in Britain looked at whether hot beverages relieved the symptoms of thirty people suffering from the flu or common cold any better than drinks at room temperature. They found that the contrast was marked.

"The hot drink provided immediate and sustained relief from symptoms of runny nose, cough, sneezing, sore throat, chilliness and tiredness," they reported, "whereas the same drink at room temperature only provided relief from symptoms of runny nose, cough and sneezing."

While this was the first study to look specifically at the effects of hot drinks on cold and flu symptoms, others have looked at hot foods like chicken soup and had similar results (chicken soup also contains cold-fighting compounds that help dissolve mucus in the lungs and suppress inflammation, as we learned in *Never Shower in a Thunderstorm*).

But what about a dose of heat on a much larger scale—say, in a sauna?

With temperatures of 176 degrees Fahrenheit (80 degrees Celsius) or greater, saunas have been recommended for arthritis, asthma, and chronic fatigue, among other things, since they were first used by nomads in Finland centuries ago. Some reputed benefits have not been examined, or are dubious at best, but there is evidence that saunas may speed recovery from colds and reduce their occurrence.

Some researchers suspect sauna heat reduces symptoms because it improves drainage, while others speculate that the high temperatures help weaken cold and flu viruses. Why this might prevent sickness in the first place, however, is unclear. But research suggests an effect.

In one study by Austrian researchers, for example, a group of fifty adults were split into two groups and tracked for six months. One group was instructed to use saunas regularly; the other group abstained. At the end of the study the sauna group had contracted fewer colds than the others. "This was found particularly during the last three months of the study period, when the incidence was roughly halved compared to controls," the scientists wrote.

A cup of hot tea, a quick spin in the sauna, and a bowl of chicken soup. Even on a wintry day when I'm feeling healthy as a horse, this combination would sound pretty good.

CAN TAKING ZINC HELP YOU BEAT A COLD?

It starts every year around the same time, its arrival signaled by a succession of telltale sounds that flow together like a symphony in four movements: the quick rustling of gathering winds, the soft trudging of feet through blankets of snow, the roar of football fans, and then, inevitably, the rising crescendo of sneezing, sniffling, and raspy coughs.

It is the onset of cold season, in the Northern Hemisphere in early December, and every year as it gets under way, countless achy, congested, Kleenex-toting people across the globe turn to the age-old remedy of zinc as their treatment of choice.

Zinc has been around long enough to have sprouted a booming industry of lozenges, nasal sprays, and other over-the-counter formulations. But when it comes down to it, zinc's cold-fighting abilities may very well be the Bigfoot of the world of cold treatments—there is plenty of talk and speculation, but not a whole lot of evidence to back it up.

More than one hundred studies in the past two decades have examined whether zinc actually works. A few have concluded that it has some effectiveness, and have proposed various reasons. But many, many more have found little or no proof that it works. Considering that no one knows exactly how zinc is supposed to ease or prevent colds, and that high doses of it for a couple of weeks or more can lead to gastrointestinal distress and other adverse events, that is no minor detail.

One of the most extensive studies appeared in the journal *Clinical and Infectious Diseases*. In it, scientists randomly assigned more than five hundred people to receive placebo or zinc lozenges in various doses. About half the subjects had natural colds, while the other half were part of a brave and growing breed of subjects in the world of scientific research: people who volunteer to be infected with cold viruses, usually by squeezing infected droplets in their noses. It's a skin-crawling procedure that is repeated in countless cold studies every year, and if you happen to be one of the people who have or will someday volunteer for this job, I salute you for your service.

In any case, while the subjects were secluded in hotel rooms and examined over a period of five days, they were assigned to take various doses of zinc gluconate, zinc acetate, or a placebo. At the end of the study, the researchers found that neither of the formulations had any effect on the duration or severity of natural cold symptoms, and they concluded that "zinc compounds appear to have little utility for common-cold treatment."

Not exactly a ringing endorsement.

Another study, published in 2007 by researchers at Stanford Medical School, collected and analyzed data from fourteen previous placebo-controlled studies of zinc. Overall, the scientists determined, the effectiveness of zinc lozenges "has yet to be established," though there was some slight evidence for zinc nasal gels. That seems to be the case with the majority of studies that look into zinc. There's plenty of proof against it, and yet, nonetheless, there remains a morsel of evidence that's tantalizing enough to keep the search going—not unlike the case with Bigfoot.

IS IT A COLD? IS IT AN ALLERGY? HOW CAN YOU TELL THE DIFFERENCE?

A stuffy head, a sore throat, and fits of sneezing so intense they could leave you with a migraine: many of us know the feeling.

These would seem to be the makings of a cold. Or, just as easily, they could also signal an allergy, especially during the spring and summer seasons.

It's a confusion that I know all too well. For years, I've suffered from occasional bouts of stuffy-headedness and congestion so bad that it felt at times as if a newspaper had been jammed into my sinuses. I always wondered why I was so prone to colds, until one balmy summer day when a friend who couldn't take my incessant, odd sneezing brought me to my senses with his characteristic pithiness: "Dude, do you have the world's worst allergies or something?"

Why hadn't I thought of that? I had never been to an allergist, and the thought of anything but a weak immunity to colds had not crossed my mind.

It turns out I'm not alone. According to surveys, one out of five Americans report experiencing symptoms like these at the same time every year. That would suggest they are due to an allergy, rather than a cold. But how can you tell the difference?

Symptoms of seasonal allergies and colds closely overlap, but studies suggest there are surefire ways to tell them apart.

The first is the onset of symptoms. Colds move more slowly, taking a day or longer to set in and gradually worsening with symptoms like loss of appetite and headache before subsiding again after about a week and disappearing within ten days.

But allergies begin immediately. The sneezing is sudden and overwhelming, not gradual, and the congestion, typically centered behind the nose, is immediate. Allergy symptoms also disappear quickly—almost as soon as the offending allergen, like pollen or ragweed, is no longer around.

Then there are hallmark symptoms of each. Allergies virtually always cause itchiness in the eyes, the nose, and the throat, while the common cold generally does not. Telltale signs of a cold are a fever, aches, and colored mucus.

Whichever affliction it is, it matters, since determining whether it's a cold or an allergy will determine what medication you need.

But if your symptoms are so murky that you remain in the dark, try consulting your family tree: studies show that if your parents both have allergies, you have a 75 percent chance of developing them too. Having just one parent with an allergy does too, particularly if that parent is your mother. Why that is, we don't yet know.

Is drinking hot water from the tap bad for you?

Decades ago, Old World chefs and cooks were routinely taught certain truths from their teachers and mothers, who in turn had learned them from the generation before, which is how we got the phrase "old wives' tale." Nowadays we have scientific studies to help us distinguish bogus tales from certain truths, but a number of questionable kitchen sayings still persist.

One of the claims that has puzzled me ever since I heard it as a twelve-year-old is the one that hot water from the tap is for washing dishes and nothing else. Drink it, the saying goes, and you risk imbibing a slew of toxins. It's a claim that has the ring of a myth, but a raft of environmental studies say it's real.

The reason is that hot water dissolves contaminants more quickly than cold water, and many pipes in homes contain levels of lead—a neurotoxin that can damage the nervous system, especially in young children—that can leach into water.

Lead is rarely found in source water, but can enter drinking water through corroded plumbing. The Environmental Protection Agency says that older homes are more likely to have lead pipes and fixtures, but that even newer plumbing advertised as "lead-free" can still contain as much as 8 percent lead. A study published in the *Journal of Environmental Health* found that tap water represented 14 to 20 percent of Americans' total lead exposure.

Scientists emphasize that the risk is small. But to minimize it, the EPA says cold tap water should always be used for preparing baby formula, cooking, and drinking. It also warns that boiling water does not remove lead but can actually increase its concentration. Something to keep in mind next time you grab a cup and reach for the tap.

Should you always cool hot leftovers at room temperature?

What to do with leftovers? Eat them, of course. But that's the easy part. Many amateur cooks—and even some expert ones—have struggled with confusion over how best to handle and store a batch of remaining portions, especially when they are still steaming or piping hot.

One common belief is that leftovers stored in a refrigerator must be allowed to cool at room temperature first, lest some major problems arise. Those who favor the cool-first approach argue that allowing food to cool at a slower rate reduces the likelihood that it will spoil. On top of that, they argue, hot food can interfere with the circulation of cold air in the refrigerator, and will force it to use more energy to cool the food, causing the machine undue strain and potentially damaging it.

That's a head scratcher. It's about the same as suggesting that putting too many hot people in an air-conditioned room will force the air conditioner to work a lot harder, making it break. The notion may have originated back when food was stored in iceboxes, and thus could not be too hot when put away. Perhaps the very people who remember using iceboxes before those newfangled refrigerators started appearing are the same ones pushing this myth.

Because whatever the rationale, the claim is wrong. According to the Food and Drug Administration, leftover food (particularly meat) should be refrigerated *immediately* after serving, and certainly within two hours of cooking. The reason is that food bacteria grow rapidly at room temperature, doubling in amount roughly every thirty or forty minutes. Several outbreaks of food poisoning have been linked to meat cooked and left to cool at room temperature for too long.

Consider what happened in Cleveland on March 18, 1993. On that day, the city health department received a rash of unusual calls from fifteen people, all of whom claimed they got sick after eating corned beef from a local deli. A newspaper published a short article about the cluster of sickness, and the health department was quickly besieged by more calls—about 160 more, in fact.

After an investigation, health authorities realized the problem: a week earlier, the deli had purchased fourteen hundred pounds of raw, salt-cured corned beef in anticipation of St. Patrick's Day. On March 12, workers at the deli cut and boiled parts of the beef for three hours, then—instead of chilling and refrigerating the food immediately—they let it cool at room temperature for some time, before finally sticking it in the refrigerator. Days later, in time for the St. Patty's celebration, the beef was removed from the refrigerator and kept in a warmer at 120 degrees Fahrenheit (48.9 degrees Celsius), so it could be sliced and used as the filling in sandwiches that were served at several catered affairs to swarms of unlucky revelers.

And there you have it, a special St. Patty's recipe that'll have you seeing red on the greenest day of the year.

Generally speaking, the bacteria that contaminate food thrive at temperatures between 40 and 140 degrees Fahrenheit (between 4.4 and 40 degrees Celsius), meaning food left out at room temperature can easily become a breeding ground. Leftovers should always be stored in a refrigerator set at 40 degrees Fahrenheit (4.4 degrees Celsius) or below. And when the quantity of food is large, it should be separated into small containers for quicker cooling, and reheated no more than once. One effective way to cool and store hot leftovers is to pack them in ziplock bags and lay them flat, which expands the food's surface area and allows its heat to escape more rapidly.

And in case you're ever tempted to save yourself some trouble and throw everything away, here are ten ways to make use of leftovers that might persuade you otherwise:

- Save them and feed to your pets.
- Turn leftover pasta into a baked casserole.
- Add to omelets or mix in with scrambled eggs for a special "Breakfast Mess."
- Use as filling for dumplings.
- Veggie scraps make great additions to soups.
- Use leftover rice to make egg or veggie fried rice the next day.
- Fruit scraps are great for yogurts, smoothies, and pies.
- Use leftover turkey from Thanksgiving to make turkey pot-pie.
- Use bread crusts to make croutons or stuffing.
- Add any leftover meats to a tortilla, then mix in some cheese, salsa, or other ingredients for flavor, and roll it up.

ARE PUBLIC RESTROOMS AS FILTHY AS EVERYONE THINKS THEY ARE?

To a germaphobe, few things are more terrifying than the dreaded public restroom. They are widely considered the most bacteria-laden places on Earth. On any given day, in almost any given restroom, we are forced to deal with dirt and grime, unbearably strong odors, footprints in strange places, and the fact that water or liquid of another sort has seemingly been splashed everywhere, and, if you happen to be in the wrong town, you may open a stall door and find a United States senator on a speed date. The conditions in any given stall are enough to test a person's bladder control and acrobatic abilities.

All of which is why I, like many hygiene-conscious Americans, approach most restrooms with as much caution as I might approach the slippery edge of a cliff. According to a nationwide survey conducted by Harris Interactive in 2008, although the vast majority of Americans use public restrooms, about 30 percent say they only use them in dire emergencies. About 70 percent of women say they have turned around and walked out of a public restroom because they decided it was "too dirty" (compared to 54 percent for men), about 55 percent of men and women said they flush the toilet with their feet, and about 19 percent of men (and 13 percent of women) said they have gone out of their way to go home and relieve themselves rather than use a public restroom.

Talk about distaste. Even Congress has higher approval ratings. (At least, most of the time.)

But how much truth does the conventional wisdom about public restrooms really hold? Over the years, various studies have flushed out an unexpected truth: they are generally not so bad, at least compared with other public areas.

One of the most extensive and revealing studies of the claim was conducted by a team of scientists at the University of Arizona and published in the *International Journal of Environmental Health Research*. The team spent four years collecting nearly eleven hundred samples at places like airports, restaurants, offices, and bathrooms in four American cities: Chicago, Tucson, San Francisco, and Tampa.

The scientists looked specifically for levels of bacteria as well as biological markers that indicated the presence of things like sweat, hemoglobin, and urea.

The most frequently contaminated areas were playgrounds and day care centers, with 46 percent showing high levels of contamination. Public restroom surfaces ranked far behind, at 25 percent, just ahead of public transportation handrails and armrests (in buses, for example) and shopping cart handles (about 21 percent each). Not far behind that were escalator handrails (19 percent), vending machine buttons (14 percent), and public phones (13 percent).

The study also found that in about 86 percent of cases, the

contaminants on a surface were transferred to an individual's hands, and then, in 82 percent of cases, to personal belongings. We know from other studies that germs are also frequently spread from one person to another via handshakes and other physical contact, and that a person can infect him- or herself by touching a germy surface and then placing that hand on the face or another vulnerable body part.

The nation's germ obsession comes as little surprise, especially in the wake of the SARS (severe acute respiratory syndrome) and avian flu epidemics, nationwide food-borne outbreaks, and the endless stream of advertisements for antibacterial products that run the gamut from hand soaps to keyboards. But at least now we know where the real risks lurk. What hasn't changed, and will always remain the same, is the most effective way to reduce the risk of spreading or contracting illness: washing your hands with plain old soap and water, which reduces your risk by 50 to 80 percent.

List of sites that were tested for the presence of protein and biochemical markers
Sample number (percentage with biochemical markers)

Shopping 333 (21 percent)
    Malls 163 (24 percent)
        Telephones, tables, handles (strollers, doorknobs, trash cans, stairs, escalators), elevator buttons, restrooms,* display cases, chairs, high-chairs, countertops
    Grocery stores 90 (17 percent)
        Telephones, shopping cart handles, food items (fruit, meat packages), refrigerator handles, common-use pens
    Vending machines 43 (14 percent)
        Newspaper, soda, food, ATM buttons, arcade games, candy machines, water machines
    Banks 28 (29 percent)
        ATM buttons, common-use pens, countertops
    Copy stores 9 (11 percent)
        Copy buttons, countertops

Activities 308 (21 percent)

Gyms 18 (28 percent)

Pool surfaces (benches, counters, locker handles), exercise equipment, handrails, water fountains, doorknobs, restrooms*

Air travel 25 (4 percent)

Armrests, food trays, luggage carts, water fountains, escalators, phones, restrooms*

Playgrounds 42 (36 percent)

Children's playground equipment (indoor and outdoor play equipment), children's rides, park surfaces (concession counters, restrooms*)

Bus travel 31 (35 percent)

Benches, handrails, call buttons, armrests, vending machines

Restaurants 51 (14 percent)

Menus, tables, table condiments, restrooms*

Doctor's offices 39 (10 percent)

Armrests, children's play areas, elevator buttons, waiting-room phones

Movie theaters 57 (26 percent)

Armrests, water fountains, restrooms,* video games, phones, doorknobs

Miscellaneous 45 (38 percent)

Parks (benches, water fountains), swimming pools (locker-room benches, tables)

Day care 54 (46 percent)

Kitchen surfaces, highchairs, toys, cups, changing tables, play tables, restrooms*

Office 105 (11 percent)

Copier buttons, computer keyboards, file-cabinet handles, phones, fax machines, doorknobs, restrooms*

Personal items 20 (5 percent)

Purses, backpacks, briefcases, home surfaces (sink, refrigerator, toys, washing machines)

---

*Faucets, doorknobs, baby changing tables, toilet flush handles and seat, soap and towel dispenser handles

CAN YOU DISINFECT A KITCHEN SPONGE BY MICROWAVING IT?

When you think of all the potential bacterial breeding grounds in a typical household, kitchen countertops do not immediately come to mind. Bathrooms, toilets, and floors, of course. But countertops—the very places we cut, prepare, and in some cases eat our food?

In fact, the kitchen sink and countertop may very well be the most unsanitary areas in many households. And all because of the kitchen sponge, that multicolored germ magnet that soaks up bacteria like, well, a sponge. Not many people realize it, but bacteria thrive on sponges, which provide them with everything they need to multiply: food, moisture, room temperatures, and a clingy surface that allows them to nest. When most people grab a moist sponge and swipe it across the counter to clean it, they are really spreading more germs than they're removing. Consider that in one study at the University of Arizona, researchers found that kitchen sponges typically harbor *E. coli*, salmonella, staphylococcus, yeasts, and molds, among other pathogens, and that two drops of liquid from a moist sponge can be loaded with as much as "10 million colony-forming units of disease-causing bacteria" that stay active for as long as two weeks. And all it takes is two days of normal use for a brand-new sponge to collect millions of pathogens.

To eliminate this emerging kitchen menace, food safety experts began encouraging people to microwave their sponges. It sounds unusual, but studies suggest it actually works. In one, published in the *Journal of Environmental Health* in 2006, scientists found that microwaving kitchen sponges and other scrubbing pads for one to two minutes at full power could reduce levels of bacteria, including *E. coli* and other common causes of food-borne illness, by more than 99 percent. Another one in 1999 found that many bacteria are eliminated within the first fifteen seconds of being heated by microwave, and that only *E. coli* survive longer than thirty seconds.

One small problem? Tossing a dry sponge in a microwave can start a fire—as evidenced by the sudden uptick in microwave-related fires across the United States after word of the disinfecting powers of microwave ovens got out. Scientists who advocate the method were suddenly deluged with calls and letters from people complaining that their kitchens nearly went up in flames. "When I put my sponge/scrubber into the microwave, it caught fire, smoked up the house, ruined my microwave, and pissed me off," one person wrote, according to MSNBC.

To avoid fires or overheating, only damp sponges and those without metal can be zapped. But some experts still argue that the practice poses a safety hazard and should be discouraged. One alternative is soaking used sponges in diluted solutions of bleach, which is just as effective as heating.

Then again, there is an even simpler option: tossing the sponge out and getting a new one.

Is it true you should never eat shellfish in a month without an R?

It is said that Native Americans introduced this warning centuries ago to early settlers, though that begs all sorts of questions about which calendar was being referred to. (The warning was actually about not eating shellfish in the summer.) But regardless, it seems the saying may be outdated.

Shellfish can be problematic in the summer months—namely May through August, none of which have an R—for several reasons. The first has to do with red tides, the vast blooms of algae that collect along coastlines, usually in warm weather. These eye-dazzling tides can spread toxins that are soaked up by oysters, clams, and mussels.

Studies have linked toxic outbreaks to this phenomenon, but only when people ate locally harvested shellfish. Most of us, however, have little reason to worry. The majority of shellfish sold in restaurants, supermarkets, and urban areas are commercially harvested, and as a result are subject to regulations intended to eliminate such hazards. The regulatory system has seen its share of failures lately—toxic toys, anyone?—but on this front it seems to be working.

Another problem in the summer is that it's usually the time of year when shellfish spawn. As any oyster aficionado knows, a fertile oyster turns unpleasantly thin, milky, and soft—far from ideal. Smarter vendors tend to avoid this problem by importing shellfish from cooler climates. Oysters can also be genetically modified so they don't spawn. But while these Franken-fish taste the same as their regular counterparts, they tend to look somewhat different, which can be off-putting to a lot of diners.

Finally, shellfish can spoil more easily on a hot day if not stored properly. While that makes them unappetizing, for sure, it doesn't necessarily make them toxic.

DOES DOUBLE-DIPPING SPREAD GERMS?

Jerry's friend George Costanza helped introduce a phrase to the national consciousness when he enraged a fellow character at a funeral reception on an episode of the television show *Seinfeld*. "Did, did you just double dip that chip?" the other man, clearly agitated and disgusted, interrogates him. "That's like putting your whole mouth right in the dip!"

As funny as the ensuing scene and George's response—"You dip the way you want to dip, I'll dip the way I want to dip"—were, the moment also instilled fear and caution at Super Bowl parties everywhere. In the mind of any germaphobe, conspicuously double-dipping any chip in a communal bowl of dip is tantamount to taking a deep swig from a bottle of white wine at a party and then handing it to the people standing behind you, empty wineglasses in hand.

But if you've ever wondered whether double-dipping is truly a bacterial hazard, or just a hazardous figment of the sitcom imagination, then science has come to the rescue with the answer. A team of scientists at Clemson University in South Carolina took the double-dipping maxim to task in 2008. Their verdict? Well, suffice it to say that from now on, you may want to opt for smaller chips that allow for a single plunge and no more, because a double-dipped chip can in fact contaminate the entire bowl.

For their study, the team had volunteers take bites of crackers and then dip their crackers for about three seconds into a test dip. There were six test dips with varying ingredients: a commercial salsa, a cheese dip, chocolate syrup, and clean water with three different levels of acidity. Each dip was exposed to either three or six double scoops, before the dip sample was analyzed to see whether it contained any bacteria. Not expecting to see much of an effect, the scientists were surprised by what they found.

A double-dip, it turns out, transferred thousands of bacteria from the offender's mouth to the dip—and about fifty to one hundred of those bacteria subsequently made their way onto a second, clean chip. If you were at a party and that clean chip was in your hand, the bacteria that hitched a ride as you plunged that chip into the dip would be destined for your mouth. As they say, bon appétit.

But there's more. The type of dip involved affected the outcome. The thicker the dip, the less likely it was to become a breeding ground, apparently because the higher viscosity forced more of a person's saliva to stay on the chip. Thinner dips allow bacteria from a double-dipper's chip to slough off and travel into the bowl.

Like viscosity, acidity also made a difference: dips with higher levels of acidity kill off more bacteria. But it won't kill all of it.

Next time you're at a party and you plunge chip into a bowl of dip, be aware that you may be swapping spit with the other guests.

The authors of the study put it another way. "Whether the amount of contamination is dangerous to the dipper's health or not is still debatable and can depend on multiple external factors including the type of chip/dip or the relative health/illness of the person whose mouth provided the bacteria," they wrote. "Next time you take a bite of your chip, and are tempted to commit a second dip, keep in mind that the numbers have been calculated, and the bacteria are having just as much of a party as you are."

IS THERE ANY TRUTH TO THE FIVE-SECOND RULE?

The five-second rule has a nice ring to it, that much is true. But I prefer another title, the no-one-saw-it rule, because if no one else saw it hit the ground, then in my book it is fair game. As an old Chinese saying goes, "Big germs eat little germs."

But despite our own personal preferences, behind the claim is a valid question: If you pick up a dropped piece of food before you can count to five, are germs really less likely to stick, making the food okay to eat? It's not difficult to imagine that bacteria on a surface would begin attaching themselves to food immediately. But how many, and does the type of surface in question make any difference?

Thank goodness we have serious scientists to put such pressing questions to the test.

As it turns out, the same team of researchers who put their

minds to the double-dipping issue conducted a rigorous laboratory study in 2007 that addressed precisely these queries. For the study, Professor Paul L. Dawson, the lead researcher, decided that his bacterium of choice would be salmonella, the all-too-common cause of food poisoning that many of us have come to know and hate.

Then, Dawson and his colleagues set out to examine several surfaces to determine how long the bacteria could survive on them. They chose tile, nylon carpet, and wood flooring. Each was lightly painted with a broth of salmonella that amounted to roughly several million bacteria per square centimeter of surface.

What they found explains something about salmonella that is more than a little disconcerting. The bacteria managed not only to survive, but thrive: after twenty-four hours, thousands remained on the tile and wood, and hundreds were still alive four weeks later. The carpet was the surface that was most conducive to survival, allowing tens of thousands of bacteria to continue living a day after the study began.

Was that a stomach growl I heard? Don't worry, there's more.

Dawson and his colleagues then dropped slices of dry food (bread) and moist food (bologna slices) on the surfaces and counted how many live bacteria the food absorbed after varying amounts of time. Tick, tick, tick. Three seconds went by. Tick, tick. Another two seconds came and went, and the researchers removed their slices and analyzed their bacterial counts.

Moisture, of course, would generally be expected to sop up the most bacteria, and by that standard the bologna did not disappoint. Over 99 percent of bacterial cells were transferred from the tile to the bologna slices after five seconds. But the transfer from carpet to bologna was quite low (less than 1 percent) compared to the transfer from wood and tile (up to 68 percent). The bread, with less moisture, was less of a bacteria magnet.

Overall, the five-second rule appeared vindicated—to some extent, that is. As the amount of time that the slices of food spent on the surfaces increased, so too did the amount of bacteria that attached to them. But considering that for some strains of salmonella it only takes as few as ten—I repeat, ten—bacteria to cause illness, the only second that might matter is the first one. That's how long it takes ten bacteria to jump from a surface to your food.

In the end, bacteria are only one part of the equation. Most floors and surfaces are also teeming with trace amounts of chemicals and surface cleaners, not to mention plain old dirt. These are all substances that you most certainly do not want to ingest.

But then, if you live in a home that has a cat or a dog, none of this will probably matter anyway. Chances are, any piece of food that hits the ground will be gone in under a second anyway.

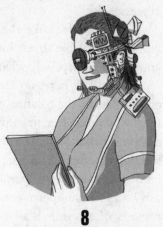

8

HI, TECHNOLOGY

Modern Life Medicine

It has taken me an inordinate amount of time to write this section, a full three days.

It's not that it's a particularly long one, or that I'm a slow writer (though some of my more prickly editors would surely beg to differ). It is more so that I have been swept up in the rogue waves of my own health-obsessed thoughts. You see, as a health reporter, the information I am often privy to—through my perusal of medical journals, obscure studies, and research databases—can be extremely useful and practical, not to mention great fodder for conversation at social gatherings. But it can also leave me hamstrung. There are times when I find my head throbbing as I contemplate completing some small, mundane chore that also carries with it some unusual hazard that I learned of in one of the millions of studies whose findings are tattooed on the part of my brain that processes risk.

At times I feel like the slaughterhouse worker who turns vegetarian, unable to eat his own company's products with the knowledge of precisely what's in them.

And so I sit here, on Day 3, with my obligations suspended on one side of the balance, and my aversion to risk on the other. Ideally I would place my aging computer on my lap and write up a storm, even though it tends to overheat and radiate only slightly less warmth than a hydrogen bomb. But then I remember the studies that discovered that placing a laptop on—where else?—the lap can lead to a low sperm count and infertility, and that even a few minutes of exposure is all it takes to do damage.

"It's simple," you're probably thinking, "just place the computer on the coffee table and lean forward."

But that, too, poses its own unique problem. Sitting at a desk or on a couch with the body hunched forward—the position we typically take when we work on a laptop that's resting on a table— produces more spinal disk movement than pretty much every other sitting position. A 90-degree posture is not much better. Those facts came to me courtesy of a groundbreaking imaging study in 2006. And with my brittle lower back, which may as well be made from glass, I take those findings seriously. But if I take a third route, perching the laptop on a small throw pillow off to my side, I risk arching my hands in a way that might heighten my risk of carpal tunnel syndrome—or so I've learned from various studies.

When it comes to even the simplest tasks, it seems, hazards are all around us. No wonder I am constantly on alert. And it's clear I'm not the only one. I know this because on the Web site of the *Times*, you can find a list of the top ten most e-mailed articles at any given time. When I write a column that delves into some kind of hidden danger, especially when it involves technology or something that exists around the household, it's sure to make that list: things like whether hot water from the tap is unsafe for cooking or if it's truly dangerous to talk on a cell phone in a hospital or in an airplane.

Plenty of people struggle to be vigilant about their health, sometimes to the point that they drive themselves mad. Perhaps you're even one of them. But the only solution is to sift through the studies, find the bottom line, and react accordingly. Some of the dangers that others overlook really are worth making into a big deal. Others aren't worth sweating. In the following pages, we'll take a look at some of the ones that are most pressing.

And if you're wondering how I ended up finishing this section, I decided that the risk of carpal tunnel syndrome was one that I could accept. Flip through to the next page, and you'll discover why.

CAN YOU STAND TOO CLOSE TO YOUR MICROWAVE OVEN?

Considering how long microwave ovens have been around, you would think that any concerns about their safety would have been resolved long ago. But many people continue to wonder whether standing next to a microwave while it's on can expose them to radiation—and if so, how much.

I have met people who eat TV dinners on a nightly basis but won't stand anywhere near a microwave while it's running unless they were fitted with a hazmat suit. On occasion I've noticed that when I, too, use a microwave, I generally wander out of the room until the beeping draws me back—perhaps because of a subconscious desire not to end up cooked as well.

But the hype surrounding microwave emissions is much ado about nothing. Although microwave ovens can in fact leak radiation, the levels that might be released from some models are fairly minute.

According to the Center for Devices and Radiological Health, a unit of the Food and Drug Administration that regulates microwave oven safety, every microwave that reaches the market must meet a requirement limiting the amount of radiation it can leak in its lifetime to 5 milliwatts per square centimeter at roughly two inches away from the oven. According to the center, that is far below the levels of radiation that have been shown to harm humans.

By comparison, the most common cell phones operate at a peak power of about 1.6 watts or less, and most studies have found no evidence linking the phones to health problems.

Manufacturers of microwave ovens are also required to line the doors of the machines with metal mesh that prevents microwaves from escaping, and to use a type of door latch that stops the production of microwaves whenever the latch is released.

Those features greatly limit exposure to levels of radiation that are already low. And since the radiation levels drop sharply with increasing distance, the levels two feet away are about one-hundredth the amount at two inches. That means that the next time your food is being nuked, you'll be just about as safe whether you stick around the kitchen or hightail it to another room.

IS IT TRUE THAT YOU SHOULD NEVER USE A CELL PHONE ON AN AIRPLANE?

I have had flight attendants shout at me for getting up to stretch my legs during drink service (sorry, next time I'll raise my hand), chastise me for using the bathroom when the seat belt sign was on (never mind that the attendant had just used the bathroom himself), and rouse me from a deep sleep and insist that I put my seat in the "upright position" in preparation for landing (I assumed that the attendant wanted me to sit up straight so I could appreciate and pay full attention to the pilot's most excellent landing skills).

But of all the brain-numbing rules and rituals that airline passengers are so callously subjected to, the one that has always irked me the most is the demand that I shut off my MP3 player or laptop during takeoff and landing. Are the airlines really telling me that a 3-ounce music player is powerful enough to bring down an 800,000-pound Boeing 747 jumbo jet? And if that is indeed the case, shouldn't Boeing and the airlines concentrate on designing aircraft that are a tad less vulnerable to the monstrous forces of my powder-blue iPod Mini?

It sounds akin to a firecracker taking down a building.

Except that in this case, the matter is a bit more complicated. The rule against electronic devices is primarily aimed at devices that transmit or receive signals, like cell phones, radios, and pagers. Airplanes are built with all sorts of radio equipment that allow, among other things, radar guidance, weather detection, and communication with ground and air traffic control. These flight control devices are designed to be sensitive enough to detect extremely weak signals emanating from far, far away. The concern is that if a passenger were speaking on a cell phone in mid-flight, the signals to and from his phone might disrupt the normal operation of the equipment in the cockpit, particularly the global positioning receivers, which are crucial to landing.

If you've ever laid your cell phone on or beside a computer tower and heard static shooting from the speakers, or had one of your FM radio stations disrupted by a CB radio from a passing car or truck, then you've experienced firsthand the effects of radio interference.

On airplanes, the navigation and flight control devices have built-in shielding, but wear and tear from repeated flights can make them vulnerable. And keep in mind that while cell phones are generally designed to have low power output, when they're operated several miles above the towers on the ground, they're forced to operate at their maximum output. It's not so much the thought of one person on a cell phone that worries airlines, but the idea of dozens of passengers all chatting away at once on phones that are sending and receiving signals.

To be sure, as of 2008, there has not been any documented crash that was unequivocally attributed to interference from a passenger's cell phone, but a team of scientists at Carnegie Mellon University who have conducted tests of the effects of cell phone signals on commercial flights says it is only a matter of time. "The data support a conclusion that continued use of portable radio frequency-emitting devices such as cell phones will, in all likelihood, someday cause an accident by interfering with critical cockpit instruments such as GPS receivers," they wrote in one study. "This much is certain: there exists a greater potential for problems than was previously believed."

As for devices that need not receive signals to function, like my puny music player or flimsy laptop, the science is still out on whether they too can cause interference. The reason they are forbidden as well is that a laptop with poor shielding, for example, could conceivably transmit enough radio energy to interfere with cockpit equipment. Again, it's not so much the threat of one device, but multiple devices all operating at once in the cabin. Because the risk of serious and potentially fatal problems caused by interference easily outweighs the need for passengers to jam out on their MP3s or play Sudoku on their portable game consoles, the airlines operate on the better-safe-than-sorry principle. (Conducting serious business on your laptop doesn't cause less interference, of course.)

There's another upside to all this. Sitting on a crowded plane can be nuisance enough. Now imagine sitting on a crowded plane with every other passenger yakking on their cell phones. With all the background noise, those cell phone talkers will have plenty of reason to up the volume on their voices, forcing you to up the volume on your MP3 player. And you might very well end up in the middle seat, sandwiched between two loudmouths with runaway tongues.

Is any of this giving you a headache?

If it is, there's more bad news. A number of airlines are considering eventually installing devices known as picocells, which act as compact mobile phone towers, on some aircraft. These devices would prevent cell phones in the cabin from interfering with equipment in the cockpit, allowing passengers to yak away. It's unclear whether aviations regulators will allow them. But the mere thought is enough to make me hope and pray that the ban on electronic devices—or at least cell phones—remains in effect.

As a matter of fact, why limit the rule to airplanes? I'd rather see it expanded to include buses, waiting rooms, movie theaters, airport terminals, sidewalks, restaurants, railroad cars, coffee shops, elevators, clothing stores . . .

WHAT ABOUT CELL PHONES IN HOSPITALS?

Okay, so cell phones can in fact have an impact on navigation and flight control equipment in airplane cockpits. But equally important are the effects that they may or may not have on medical equipment, especially ventilators, heart monitors, and other machines that can mean the difference between life and death.

If you've ever absentmindedly whipped out a cell phone in a hospital, you may have found out how seriously many doctors and nurses take this rule. As an intern working in a hospital one summer back in college, I once made the mistake of pulling out my cell phone to look at the time as I was walking down a hall toward the maternity ward. A surgeon I had previously never met rapidly blew a fuse when he spotted me.

"Hey, shut that thing off!" he snapped. "Are you trying to *kill* somebody!"

Sheepishly sliding my phone back into my pocket, I slinked away and licked my wounds. It could have been a lot worse. I could have been arrested, as was the case in 1998 when a man in Wareham, Massachusetts, was pepper-sprayed in a hospital by police when he refused to stop chatting on his cell phone. According to police, the man was lying on a gurney being treated for a foot injury—he had been admitted after he kicked a fish tank while arguing with his girlfriend—and refused to follow orders from an officer and a paramedic that he get off the phone.

"Shut up, man, I'm talking to my dad in Connecticut," he responded, as quoted in the police report.

A struggle ensued, and the officer sprayed the disorderly patient—twice—then arrested him and hauled him off to jail.

I am thankful that I only suffered some humiliation and not much else. But now, having reported on all the facts, albeit years later, I almost wish I could go back to that doctor and explain that while his intentions were well-meaning, the danger that concerned him may have been inflated.

After years of widespread bans on cell phones in hospitals around the globe, the Mayo Clinic finally decided, in 2007, to carry out a detailed analysis of the claim. Perhaps there were just one too many cases of preoccupied interns strolling through the hospital's halls with cell phones in hand. Whatever the reason, scientists at the famed clinic spent a month testing sixteen different medical devices by holding cell phones next to them and rotating the phones as calls were received. The phones—common models like BlackBerrys, Nokias, Motorolas, and Sanyos—were placed near sites on the devices that are most susceptible to interference, like cable connection ports, displays, and serial ports.

The scientists found that there was interference about 44 percent of the time, and that it was usually noise interference that affected electrocardiographic and electroencephalographic machines. But the interference only occurred when the phone was within thirty-two inches of the devices, and ultimately there was never any "clinically important" interference when the phones were used in a "normal" way.

Translation: if you're on a phone and you're standing more than three feet from a medical device, there shouldn't be any problem.

But in other countries, that may not be the case. In another investigation in 2007, scientists in the Netherlands carried out a similar series of tests at the University of Amsterdam's Academic Medical Center. Rather than using actual cell phones, they employed special generators that mimicked maximum mobile phone power signals. Testing the signals' effects on sixty-one medical devices, they found that twenty-six, or about 43 percent, experienced interference. And they did not consider the disruptions minor; instead they said that most of the interference was "significant" or "hazardous" enough to directly affect patients or distract doctors.

Like the American researchers, they found that the interference generally occurred only within three feet of the medical devices. But one difference was that the Dutch researchers used a signal strength of 2 watts, which is roughly three times more powerful than the 600-milliwatt output that most phones in the United States are capable of.

So why not just ban cell phones in all hospitals according to the same better-safe-than-sorry principle employed by the airplanes? Well, it's not hard to imagine that the average hospital patient or their relatives might typically have more pressing calls to make—emergency calls to family members, for example, about a patient's rapidly diminishing condition—than the average passenger sitting on an airplane waiting for takeoff. It's also become increasingly common for doctors to conduct some aspects of their jobs by cell phone.

As things stand now, if an accident victim is in extremely

critical condition with his or her vital signs slowly dwindling and that person's mother, husband, or children need to know, then it may not be such a crime for someone to step into the hall and make an emergency call. From what the science tells us, chances are it'd be worth the risk.

IS HOSPITAL CARE WORSE ON WEEKENDS?

We all know that many public services are less reliable on weekends—government offices are shut, trains and buses run less frequently, and the ever-vigilant postman takes a day off. It's just a fact of life, one we learn to live with. But it might surprise you to hear that it seems this applies to our hospitals as well.

Not to stir too many worries, but there's good evidence from a number of studies in recent years that if you check into a hospital with a serious illness on a Saturday or Sunday, your odds of checking out—or recovering at a decent rate—are not quite as good as they would be on a Monday or Thursday. And the reason may have more to do with staffing changes than with doctors zoning out.

Most of what we know about this phenomenon comes from studies on people who suffer heart attacks—always a popular subject. In one of the largest studies, published in 2007 in the *New England Journal of Medicine*, scientists followed nearly a quarter of a million heart attack patients who were admitted to New Jersey hospitals between 1987 and 2002. They found that those who checked in on weekends suffered death rates that were a percentage point higher than those who went in on a weekday, 12.9 percent for weekend patients versus 12 percent for weekday patients. One percentage point may not sound like much, but when the sample size is nearly a quarter of a million people, that translates to a heck of a lot of deaths. (More than two thousand, and you wouldn't want to be one of them.)

After further analysis, it appeared that the gap had a lot to do with weekend patients being less likely to receive aggressive treatment. The most skilled and senior doctors often don't work weekends, and the staff that do are not as likely to perform more advanced, lifesaving operations. The researchers found, for example, that 10 percent of the weekday heart patients underwent angioplasty operations to clear blocked arteries on the day they checked in, while only 6.7 percent of weekend patients underwent the operation on their first day. A major procedure that can stop a heart attack in its tracks, angioplasty is most effective when administered within ninety minutes of the beginning of the attack.

Lest you think this applies only to heart attack patients or to emergency rooms, other scientists have found otherwise. One extensive study published in the *Annals of Surgery* in 2007, for example, looked at 188,212 patients who had elective, or nonemergency, surgeries and found that those who had their operations on a Friday and spent the weekend recovering on a regular hospital floor were 17 percent more likely to die in the following thirty days than those who had their operations earlier in the week.

So is it all the medical community's fault? There are some critics who would say no. Patients who show up on weekends may simply be sicker, these critics say, perhaps because they are the patients who brush aside symptoms and delay seeking care until the very last minute.

It is certainly possible, but the reality is that there's little evidence to support this notion. So far the studies point to staffing changes and treatment decisions as the culprits. Either way, many hospitals concede there's a lot of room for improvement. In the meantime, never put off seeing a doctor if a problem arises over the weekend—nothing is worse than no treatment at all.

Do computer keyboards cause carpal tunnel syndrome?

Anyone who has ever spent long hours in the office, tethered to a keyboard as the morning turns to afternoon and the afternoon turns to night, has heard the warnings about the perils of too much typing. Spend your days at the keyboard, the saying goes, and you're bound to end up with a near-permanent wrist splint. It is the battle scar of that well-known breed of worker, the type that cannot break free of the terminal, and inevitably is saddled with carpal tunnel syndrome, the nerve condition that strikes the hands and wrists.

It would seem to be an obvious connection. The condition occurs when the median nerve that passes through the carpal tunnel, a narrow channel in the wrist, is severely and repeatedly compressed, which over time disrupts the transmission of nerve signals. But studies over the years have found that carpal tunnel is not limited to office dwellers, and in fact may very well be more prevalent in *other* industries.

First off, it turns out that those who are at greatest risk of developing the condition are women. They suffer from it at three times the rate that men do, most likely because the carpal tunnel in women is generally three times smaller. But it also turns out that the condition is also about three times more common among assembly-line workers—including manufacturers and people who pack meat, poultry, and fish—than it is among office workers. That may be a result of the enormous weight and pressure placed on their hands daily, along with the constant bending of their wrists.

Some researchers have even questioned whether keyboards increase the risk of carpal tunnel at all. A good example is a study in 2001 by scientists at the Mayo Clinic. In it, the researchers looked at 181 office workers, most of them women, and found that 30 percent complained of numbness and tingling in their fingers, which are early signs of carpal tunnel. Of these employees, about 3.5 percent met the diagnostic criteria for the syndrome. The authors concluded that since the prevalence of carpal tunnel in the general population is also 3.5 percent, frequent computer usage does not heighten the risk of developing the syndrome.

But critics have relentlessly criticized this study and others like it. They have complained that the prevalence rate of 3.5 percent for the general population is based on outdated numbers and should be lower, and that the study did not account for age. The workers in the Mayo Clinic study were an average of forty-one years old, while many cases of carpal tunnel syndrome in the general population are not diagnosed until much later on. That means that the workers in the study who were experiencing numbness and tingling in their hands had early symptoms, and were apparently well on their way to developing carpal tunnel syndrome at the peak age of prevalence.

Either way, we can at least say that carpal tunnel syndrome is not limited to one industry, and may very well be the battle scar of another breed of worker, the heavy-duty lifter.

DOES COLD WATER BOIL MORE QUICKLY THAN HOT WATER?

As much as I tried to wrap my head around the idea that a pot of cold tap water will boil more quickly than a pot of warm water, it never made much sense. But it must have its roots in the fact that you should never drink hot water from the tap, as we saw in chapter 7. It seemed obvious that this idea about boiling times was just a stealth way to encourage people to cook with cold water, not hot, in order to avoid impurities. Another reason might be the fact that cold water gains heat at a more rapid rate than water that is already warm, though it will not boil faster under normal circumstances.

But here's where things get bizarre and counterintuitive. Under the right set of parameters, the reverse phenomenon can occur, in which a container of hot water will freeze more quickly than a container of cold water. Need a second to soak that in again? That's right—hot water turning to ice more quickly than cold water!

It's not a new phenomenon. Scientists have been trying to explain it for centuries. Aristotle may have been the first on record to describe it when he wrote the following in 350 B.C.: "If water has been previously heated, this contributes to the rapidity with which it freezes: for it cools more quickly," he wrote. "Thus so many people when they want to cool water quickly first stand it in the sun: and the inhabitants of Pontus when they encamp on the ice to fish . . . pour hot water on their rods because it freezes quicker, using the ice like solder to fix their rods." Aristotle's observation was followed by similar ones from Francis Bacon and René Descartes.

But none of these men won the glory for describing this effect. Instead, that honor went to Erasto B. Mpemba, a secondary school student from Tanzania who noticed it in 1963 while using boiled milk to make ice cream and subsequently reintroduced the concept to the scientific literature. Mpemba realized that every time he took two similar containers with identical volumes of sugary water—one at 95 degrees Fahrenheit (35 degrees Celsius) and the other at 212 degrees Fahrenheit (100 degrees Celsius)—and refrigerated them, the warmer container of water always froze first.

Today we know this as the Mpemba effect, but there are numerous reasons behind it. According to a study published in the *American Journal of Physics* in 2006, one of the primary reasons is that hot water loses mass to evaporation, so a body of hot water that is the same volume as a body of cold water will, over time, lose mass, which increases the rate at which it freezes. Less mass, less time to freeze. It's the same reason a small pond will freeze faster than a lake.

Another explanation, set out in the journal *Physics*, has to do with solutes. Most drinking water contains compounds like calcium and magnesium bicarbonate that precipitate out when the water is heated, making it easier for the water to freeze. Water that has not been heated (and whose solutes have not been precipitated out) must actually reach a lower temperature before it freezes, just as adding salt to a pot of water raises its boiling temperature. Solutes decrease freezing temperatures and have the opposite effect on boiling temperatures.

But that's not all. About a half dozen other factors in the process have been proposed, including the action of convection: colder water freezes from the top down, slowing the loss of heat from the top of the water, while hot water freezes from the bottom up because of convection currents. Some of these other explanations are a bit suspect, but it's clear that the combination of two or more of these processes can account for the effect.

So the next time you get an itch to make ice cream, follow the Mpemba effect.

WHAT'S THE SAFEST SEAT IN A CAR?

Automobiles may not be the safest mode of transport, but many people wonder whether where they choose to sit can improve their odds in an accident.

Unfortunately, as many of us know from being forced and prodded into eating our greens at the dinner table as small children, what's best for us isn't always what's most palatable. And the same applies here. Think of the seat that's least desirable, least comfortable. The seat with little room and no headrest. The one that sometimes lacks even a functional seat belt.

It's the rear middle seat, the one that the saddest soul in a full car gets stuck with. It may be the least desirable seat in any four-door car, but it turns out it's also the one that will offer the most protection in a crash and improve your odds of escaping unharmed. Uncomfortable, yes, but it's the seat that typically has the largest "crush zone," an area around which the car collapses in a collision, ultimately protecting the person filling the seat.

The largest study of the subject, conducted by researchers at the University of Buffalo in 2006, analyzed more than sixty thousand fatal crashes and found that passengers in the middle backseat were between 59 percent and 86 percent more likely to survive than those in the front seats, and 25 percent more likely to survive than those in the other rear seats. They reached that conclusion after analyzing two sets of data from the National Highway Traffic Safety Administration. One involved car crashes in which there were occupants in both the front seats and backseats, and the other involved survival rates of backseat occupants in crashes that resulted in at least one fatality.

One startling finding was that about half of all adults in the middle backseat neglected to wear seat belts. Those who refused to click it, as they say, were about three times as likely to die in a crash as middle-backseat passengers who did buckle up. But not wearing a seat belt in the back can have unfortunate consequences for those up front as well. Other scientists have found that even when passengers in the front do wear seat belts, their odds of dying are five times as great if those in the back are not belted in—a result of backseat passengers being thrown forward on impact. More reason to encourage friends who are going for a ride with you to buckle up.

Besides the security of sitting in the crush zone, people who snag the rear middle seat have improved odds for another reason. According to experts at the highway traffic safety administration, in rollover crashes, people in the rear middle are less exposed to rotational force than the people sitting next to them. It's practically a cocoon of safety. But that's only if you're strapped in.

It's enough to lead me to a new resolution: the next time I

hop in a car with a group of friends, I'm calling dibs on the middle backseat. I'd advise you to do the same.

DO SOME PEOPLE DREAM IN BLACK AND WHITE?

In an age of high-definition television and vivid cinematography, it might seem peculiar to think that anyone would experience colorless dreams.

For many people, the dream state can be the most turbulent, emotionally intense part of the day. Falling, flying, failing exams, and being chased are among the most frequently reported themes when people are asked in studies to describe their dreams. And yet for a small segment of the population, drifting off at night means reverting to an old-fashioned world of monochromatic hues.

Childhood exposure to black-and-white television seems to be the common denominator. A study published this year, for example, found that people twenty-five years old and younger say they almost never dream in black and white. But people over the age of fifty-five who grew up with little access to color television—particularly when they were between the ages of three and eleven—reported dreaming in black and white about a quarter of the time. Overall, 12 percent of people dream entirely in black and white.

Go back a half century, and television's impact on our closed-eye experiences becomes even clearer. In the 1940s, just before color televisions became commercially available, studies showed that three-quarters of Americans, including college students, reported "rarely" or "never" seeing any color in their dreams. Now, those numbers are reversed.

Perhaps fifty years from now there will be another divide, between people who merely dream in color, and those who dream in high definition.

An obvious question in all of this is why the strong connection between dreams and television? After all, we spend all of our waking hours in color. Shouldn't we spend our sleeping hours in color too?

One would think so. But apparently the connection exists because watching television and cinema can be such an emotional, adrenaline-fueled experience that it heightens our senses. It's well known that people are more likely to remember something if the occasion is fraught with emotion—anger, fear, or anxiety, for example. These heightened states can reinforce memories, which then come back to us when we shut our eyes and step into the emotionally acute world of dreams.

But what about blind people, or the colorblind? Their dreams are just as intriguing. Studies show that people born without the ability to see report no visual images in their dreams, but they may be experiencing a heightening of other senses, like taste and smell. People who become blind after the age of five rarely experience visual imagery in their dreams, although there are reports of children who lost their vision in their first five years seeing images in their dreams later on. Most people who lose their vision after age five, meanwhile, continue to see visual imagery, although the clarity may fade over time.

As for the color-blind, some people have only red-green or blue-yellow color blindness, and they dream accordingly. Complete color blindness is typically a genetic condition, something people are born with, so those who have it generally would have only experienced monochromatic hues in their waking lives, and as a result, monochromatic hues in their sleeping lives.

That said, happy dreaming.

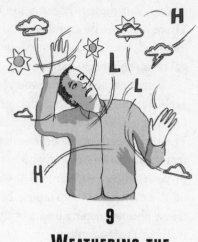

9

WEATHERING THE ELEMENTS

The Active Life

Most people love Mother Nature. But for me, the relationship is not so friendly. I constantly extend an open hand in an attempt to get along, but in return I am snubbed, my hand pushed away with extreme prejudice. Mother Nature seems to go to great lengths to let me know that I am most unwelcome, tormenting me until I flee in horror, much like the ghosts of *Poltergeist* chasing the naïve new tenants out of their home. Except no matter how insufferable the persecution, I keep returning to the house, hoping that if I stick around just long enough, Mother Nature will give up her ghastly torment and relent, allowing me to throw my feet up on the couch.

Of course, to no avail. I get the feeling I will always be treated with the sort of intense disdain usually reserved for people who honk their horns in traffic jams or loudly sing off-key in public as they listen to their CD or MP3 players. It is not a good feeling. But there is consolation in knowing that I am not alone. There seems to be a small contingent of people out there, myself included, who are shown no love. We are Mother Nature's prodigal children, her punish-worthy misfits.

These are the people who respond with knowing nods when I talk about how much suffering I routinely endure at the hands (or stingers, I should say) of mosquitoes each and every summer. Their ears perk up when I wonder aloud exactly how to escape this misfortune (will eating garlic keep those pesky bugs away—or perhaps some vitamin B?). Or they follow up with questions of their own about escaping bees and other winged attackers. (How about jumping into a body of water? And why on Earth is it so hard to swat them?)

But Mother Nature's wrath comes in many forms. If you've ever taken a trip to the beach, sprawled out on the sand, and noticed others luxuriating in the sunlight as if being wrapped in God's warmest blanket while you—perched only a few feet away—get the feeling that there's a massive magnifying glass between you and the sun, then you may be in this select group. These are the people who splurge on the most expensive suntan lotions, but wonder whether the extremely high SPF makes any difference. Or, like me, wonder whether darker skin better protects against skin cancer. Or if unusual weather patterns are responsible for our sickness.

If you've ever found yourself cursed by nature, then the following insights and explanations will resonate. Or, if you're one of the lucky ones—the favored sons and daughters—then you'll gain some insight into the plight of the unlucky few.

Does darker skin better protect you against skin cancer?

It's well known that people with darker skin get deeper tans and burn less quickly than their paler counterparts. The extra melanin acts almost something like a built-in layer of sun blocking protection—except it's not nearly as effective as one would think.

Although people with darker skin tones face a lower risk of skin cancer, they are far more likely to develop more aggressive forms of the disease and more likely to die from it. A large part of the problem is a false sense of security. Dark skin has higher amounts of melanin that can filter as much as twice the amount of ultraviolet radiation as paler skin. But that protection still falls short of what doctors recommend when using sunscreen: a skin protection factor, or SPF, of 15 or more. And because many people with dark skin believe that it provides complete immunity, experts say, they often overlook early warning signs.

A 2006 study in the *Archives of Internal Medicine* looked at more than fifteen hundred people with melanoma. It found that whites were far less likely to have late-stage melanoma than blacks, Hispanics, American Indians, and Asians. On average, whites also had a greater five-year survival rate (90 percent) than the others (less than 80 percent). Meanwhile, another study in the *Archives of Dermatology* that looked at seventeen hundred cases of melanoma that were diagnosed in Florida over a five-year period showed the same pattern.

All of this plays into a larger, unfortunate problem: most people are lax on the matter of protecting themselves from the sun's harmful rays. According to a survey by the American Academy of Dermatology in 2003, only 47 percent of women and 33 percent of men regularly use sunscreen—and even fewer know how to use it properly. In part, that's because as simple as SPF ratings and application instructions should be, they are often misleading or incomplete, as we're about to find out . . .

ARE HIGH SPF RATINGS REALLY BETTER?

Everyone knows that an SPF rating of 60 provides double the protection of SPF 30, right? Wrong. Studies over the years have shown that sunscreen with an SPF of 30 blocks about 97 percent of ultraviolet rays. A rating of 15 means 93 percent of UV rays are deflected, and anything higher than 30 remains in the 97 or 98 percent range.

In 1999 the Food and Drug Administration recommended that sunscreens with an SPF higher than 30 be labeled "30+," mostly to prevent people from developing a false sense of security that might lead them to spend more time in the sun.

What many people also fail to realize is that the amount of sunscreen applied to the skin plays an enormous role. A study in the *British Journal of Dermatology* this year found that applying less than 2 ounces over the entire body at one time can leave people with an SPF rating far lower than what is on the bottle. Some studies have shown that people typically apply just 10 percent of the amount recommended. It is also important to look for sunscreens that protect against both UVA and UVB radiation. SPF ratings apply only to UVB rays, and some sunscreens provide no protection at all against UVA rays, which penetrate the skin more deeply. For broad protection, look for sunscreens with avobenzone, zinc oxide, or titanium dioxide, all of which block UVA.

And remember some of the life advice proffered by Mary Schmich, a columnist for the *Chicago Tribune*, in a now famous column published in 1997 (and often wrongly credited to the future-looking novelist Kurt Vonnegut): "Do one thing every day that scares you. . . . Dance, even if you have nowhere to do it but your living room. . . . Get to know your parents. You never know when they'll be gone for good." And, most important, she wrote: "Wear sunscreen."

CAN THE CHLORINE IN POOLS CAUSE HAIR LOSS?

A long, vigorous swim may be good for your heart, but scientists have long questioned whether the high levels of chlorine in many swimming pools can have some less desirable effects on your hair and skin.

Swimmers are known to complain that too much time in the pool leaves their hair thin and brittle, and in some cases changes the color entirely. Many people may remember that in 2003, Scott Peterson, the California man accused of killing his wife, used that explanation when he was captured by police near the Mexican border. His hair and goatee had turned from dark to blond not because he had dyed it to evade the authorities, he said, but because he had been swimming in a neighbor's swimming pool.

Sure.

Alibis notwithstanding (Peterson was promptly arrested and later convicted), studies have found that the local pool can in fact have some pernicious effects on hair.

One of several studies on the topic was published in 2000 in the journal *Dermatology*. In that study, a team of researchers examined sixty-seven professional swimmers and fifty-four nonswimmers and found that 61 percent of the swimmers showed signs of hair discoloration, compared with none of the nonswimmers. Dark hair turns lighter, and blond hair turns green—not from the chlorine, but from another dissolved metal, in this case, copper.

In the 2000 study, scientists found that the hair discoloration coincided with surface damage of the swimmers' cuticles and nail plates, apparently due to friction with water. But although the swimmers' hair appeared coarse and damaged, they did not have higher rates of hair loss.

Pools, it seems, can act like a giant vat of dye. And not simply when it comes to hair. An unusual study by dentists in 2000 compared a group of 171 competitive swimmers to a group of 233 nonswimmer athletes. The dentists looked specifically at the subjects' teeth, finding that 60 percent of the swimmers had significant dental staining, compared to only 13 percent of the nonswimmers. After adjusting for variables like age, gender, and daily consumption of coffee and red wine, the study concluded that six hours a week of swimming is enough to create "a high risk" of dental stains. Why these dentists were compelled to study teeth and swimming may never be known (perhaps the lead author owned a pool?), but the findings are at the very least instructive.

In any case, for those worried about the effects their swimming routines may have on their appearance, consider using chlorine-removing shampoos and conditioners, which can partly avert changes in hair color. It can also help to wear a swim cap—and, perhaps, a mouth guard.

CAN EATING GARLIC WARD OFF MOSQUITOES? WHAT ABOUT VITAMIN B?

How nice it would be if eating one simple food could bring relief to all those Americans who become walking bait for mosquitoes each summer.

Garlic, perhaps because of its strong odor, has long been said to be that magic food. Another pervasive claim is that taking vitamin B—or wearing patches infused with it—can make mosquito magnets like myself all but invisible to the pests. Supposedly vitamin B releases a strong odor that mosquitoes find repugnant.

On a balmy summer day, mosquitoes pounce on me like vultures on a corpse. To say they attack me is to say a tornado is an air current; it does not begin to tell the full story. Scientifically speaking, it's not that my blood is any sweeter than that of my bite-resistant peers, it's just that some people lack the genes that produce compounds capable of masking their smell and other signals that mosquitoes home in on, as we learned in *Never Shower in a Thunderstorm*. Which is why I set out on a hunt for the remedy to my lifelong friction with mosquitoes. What food would produce the subtle odor that could finally, once and for all, get them off my back?

Garlic was first on my list. So I sifted through a mound of studies, scoured the medical databases, and talked to the entomologists who study such things. In my quest I found a study conducted in 2005 at the University of Connecticut Health Center. In it, a team of scientists asked groups of subjects to consume large amounts of garlic on some days and a placebo on others. Then, in a move that would send me running for the hills, they exposed these unfortunate subjects to swarms of mosquitoes. The number of mosquitoes that fed on the subjects and the number of bites they suffered did not seem to differ under the two conditions.

Translation: eating garlic may repel other humans, but apparently not mosquitoes.

My skin crawling, and with garlic now out of the question, I moved on to vitamin B. Surely it must produce some sort of effect, I thought, or all those advertisements for pills and patches that flood the Internet were less than truthful. Take small doses of the supplement three times a day during biting season, the ads say, and mosquitoes will give you the cold shoulder.

Sounds simple enough. But studies that have put this strategy to the test have proclaimed it a myth. In the most prominent, published in the *Journal of the American Mosquito Control Association* in 2005, scientists had a group of subjects ingest vitamin B supplements every day for eight weeks. A second ingested vitamin C, and a third took no supplements at all. Once every two weeks, packs of bloodthirsty mosquitoes were unleashed to reveal whether the supplements were having any effect. Although each subject's attractiveness varied considerably, overall there was no evidence that vitamin B did anything to help.

Another study by scientists in Brazil, where the claim is also widespread, particularly in the country's sweltering tropical jungles, examined the effects of vitamin B by having animals consume it in droplet form. When the animals were subsequently exposed to female mosquitoes (the only ones that bite), there was no difference in attractiveness between the vitamin B group and a control group that was not given the vitamin. Mosquitoes 2, edible repellents 0.

But here's the kicker. Just about the only food or beverage that has been shown to have an effect on mosquitoes when ingested by humans is alcohol: it attracts them.

In another *Journal of the American Mosquito Control Association* study, a group of fourteen subjects drank 350 milliliters of beer on various occasions. Ingesting beer significantly increased the percentage of mosquitoes that landed on the subjects, though precisely why was unclear.

What we know for certain is that mosquitoes locate their victims by seeking out body heat, lactic acid, and carbon dioxide. Alcohol may heighten your attractiveness by ramping up your output of one or all of these variables. In the end, the only substance that seems to work exceptionally well at blocking a mosquito's powers of detection—effectively disguising you—is DEET, which acts by blinding its senses. Sprays with even small amounts of the substance have been shown to work for as long as five hours. And as an added benefit, using it does not require a breath mint.

WHY IS IT SO HARD TO SWAT A FLY?

Anyone who has spent time with me in the summer knows that for me, it is the season of suffering.

In fact, I've always had an inkling that one of my good friends and college roommates used to look forward to me coming home on hot, muggy days—in part because it meant someone to crack open an ice cold beer with, but also because it meant that all the flies and mosquitoes that pestered him during the day would now have a much more appetizing target. As I've pointed out, it's a scientific fact that mosquitoes prefer some people more than others, and to them I happen to be a favorite food.

I have tried every spray and repellent known to mankind—DEET, citronella, eucalyptus—but each one has its drawbacks, and none is nearly as fulfilling as squashing a bloodthirsty mosquito with a well-timed whack. But like most people, I find myself having about as much success hitting a mosquito as I might have if I tried to make rope out of sand.

Desperate, frustrated, and tired of swinging my arms around in vain, I decided to call up someone who could help me and perhaps, in turn, millions of others like me around the globe. The man I reached was Michael Dickinson, a bioengineering professor at the California Institute of Technology. Dickinson is about as "fly" as they come: he has spent the last twenty years studying the neurobiology and biomechanics of flies. He built a tiny robotic fly called Robofly, he uses high-tech cameras to analyze the flight of winged insects, and his e-mail address pretty much says it all: flyman@caltech.edu.

So, I begged to know, why is it so hard to successfully swat a fly or a mosquito? Well, his answer came: they can pretty much see my futile swipes coming a mile away, and their brains are wired to avoid it.

Dickinson knows this because in 2008 he carried out a study that used high-speed cameras to examine how a fly reacts as it detects a threat, like the presence of an agitated science writer. At the mere hint of such a threat, the fly reacts within milliseconds. "What we used to think flies did when they saw a threatening stimulus was quickly pull the trigger and jump in the air as fast as they could," Dickinson told me. "But we found that long before the fly jumps, it actually plans its escape route. It performs what amounts to fancy footwork to position its legs and body such that when it does eventually jump, it will push itself away from the oncoming predator or swatter."

In other words, the fly calculates where and from what angle a person's hand might be coming—from the front, behind, or side, for example—and it uses that information to shift into a stance that will allow it to escape in the opposite direction, clearing the way for a successful getaway. Flies have six legs, and use their middle legs to jump off into flight. If the fly decides a swat will come from behind, for example, it shifts its middle legs in the other direction, leans forward, and readies for a forward takeoff. These preflight movements take place at least a tenth of a second before the fly actually needs to jump.

"It's premotor planning, which is a rather sophisticated form of behavior," Dickinson said.

Imagine a boxer ducking off to the side just as his opponent starts to throw his arm back and wind up for a left hook, and that begins to explain the sophisticated manner in which flies react. It also helps explain why, on every occasion that I swat furiously at a fly or mosquito that lands on my arm, I end up with a swollen red arm and not much else.

But now that we know their escape strategies, we can strike

more judiciously. "The key is to anticipate that the fly is going to jump away from the swatter, so instead of swatting where you see it, you'd want to swat a little bit opposite from the direction of your swatter," Dickinson said. "So you basically want to lead the fly. You shouldn't swat where the fly is resting, you should swat where the fly is going to head when it takes off."

Simply put, don't aim for the insect's exact spot, aim for the spot just ahead or behind it—whichever direction it seems most likely to take, since it's already leaning in that direction and is much quicker than you or me. The other good news is that this should pretty much apply to all insects, whether they bite or not, Dickinson said.

Our days of futile swipes and endless itching may be coming to an end.

CAN YOU ESCAPE A SWARM OF BEES BY JUMPING INTO A BODY OF WATER?

If you've ever been stung by a honeybee—especially in a sensitive area, like the eyes or your head—then you know it's a pain you want to avoid suffering again at all costs.

For years, I was told that I could avoid another sting by wearing light clothes. Honeybees always seek out dark clothes, I was told, so dress like you're leading a college tour group.

Didn't work. My first week at summer camp one year, I had a honeybee go straight for my khaki shorts and another one attack me so viciously I thought it would end up ripping the white polo shirt off my back like it was Hulk Hogan. I'm not a big cologne guy and my deodorants are always unscented, so it couldn't have been my odors that attracted them and the other bees that seem to become enraged anytime I so much as even drive past a camping ground.

Over time, I was instructed by multiple outdoorsy types, and even a few camping guidebooks, that one surefire way to escape a gang of bees is to jump into a body of water. Bees are pretty determined, I was told, but even the most aggressive ones can't swim, and they'll back off and reverse course if you disappear under water for a few brief moments.

Although I surely would've given it a shot, the need to do so thankfully never did arise.

Not that it matters. These days I've added that escape strategy to my "waste-of-time" list.

After consulting several bee education centers, I learned that on a scale of effectiveness, this method ranks only slightly ahead of pretending to be invisible. Bees, if irritated enough, will follow you to the body of water and easily wait for at least fifteen minutes—obviously too long to hold your breath under water, as the magician and endurance artist David Blaine can attest (his record: seven minutes, eight seconds).

The Department of Agriculture, in conjunction with the Carl Hayden Bee Research Center, put it this way: "Do not jump into water! The bees will wait for you to come up for air."

I believe there's only one way to interpret that. So what *can* you do if attacked by a swarm of bees?

Well, it's pretty simple really: run for your life.

Unlike an encounter with a grizzly bear, playing dead won't work. But humans can run faster than bees can fly. According to the Department of Agriculture, it's best to run until you reach an enclosed space, like a car or a building, and shut yourself in. Once inside, cover up with whatever is available—blankets, clothes, towels—taking special care to protect your eyes, head, and any other particularly sensitive area. If any bees have managed to slip inside before you shut the door, they will likely give up after twenty minutes at most, especially if there are windows inside, since bees tend to grow confused by well-lit areas and will gravitate toward windows. After waiting it out a little while, you should be able to safely slip out.

If for some reason you do end up getting stung a couple of times, keep the following in mind: the average person can safely tolerate more than eleven hundred stings. Not that you'd want to give it a try.

DOES A PERSON STRUCK BY LIGHTNING RETAIN AN ELECTRICAL CHARGE?

For some reason we tend to think of a person who has recently been electrocuted as a human live-wire, a downed power line ready to send electricity surging through any person unfortunate enough to help out.

It may be fit for a movie, but it's not reality. A person who has been shocked or electrocuted can be unsafe to touch, but not if the cause is a lightning strike.

It is a popular misconception that lightning is conducted through people, but experts say it stems from a different electrical phenomenon. Ron Holle, a former meteorologist who tracks lightning injuries, said that when a person is shocked or electrocuted by an exposed wire or electrified plate, those who try to help the victim are often electrocuted as well. But that only happens when the victim is still attached to the wire or electrical object.

Without that object conducting electricity, no current will flow from the victim to the rescuer. Since a typical lightning strike lasts only a few tenths of a second, this isn't a concern after a lightning strike. The human body isn't a battery; it doesn't store electricity, so administering first aid or CPR to a lightning-strike victim is perfectly safe. "Sometimes in the panic of the situation," Holle says, "people have these lingering questions." But there's no reason for them.

Another popular misconception is that it's safe to be in a car during a lightning storm because rubber tires act as an insulator. Most cars do protect against lightning, but the reason is that the metal roof and sides act as a cage that conducts electricity around the occupants. The rubber tires have nothing to do with the protection from lightning, although sometimes when a car is struck, a tire or two might explode as the electricity arcs from the car to the ground.

And people who think they're safe in a thunderstorm as long as they stay on their bicycles or motorcycles (or in their open convertibles) are wrong.

Some other shocking facts about lightning you probably didn't know:

- The average lightning bolt packs 100,000,000 volts, while the average electrical outlet produces only 110 volts, and the average electrical appliance carries only 10 amps.
- Rwanda is the lightning capital of the world, experiencing on average a staggering 82.7 lightning flashes per square kilometer. That is 2.5 times the amount of lighting that strikes the lightning capital of the United States, central Florida.
- The majority of the 326 people who were killed in lightning strikes in Florida between 1951 and 1991 died in open fields (45 percent) and under trees (23 percent).
- Between fifty and one hundred cloud-to-ground lightning bolts strike the planet every second.
- The temperature of a typical lightning bolt is hotter than the surface of the Sun!
- The diameter of a typical lightning bolt is less than that of a half-dollar. It only looks wider because the flash is so intense.

CAN THUNDERSTORMS CAUSE
ASTHMA ATTACKS?

Most people know that smoke, mold, and allergens in the air can set off an asthma attack. But thunderstorms?

It is something I had never thought of until a reader of the *New York Times*—sensing my interest in stormy weather—brought it to my attention. I am someone who struggled with asthma for years as a child, and yet the notion that stormy weather may have been the cause of my suffering seemed, when I was asked about this, too fantastical to believe.

But having investigated countless claims that sounded at first like myth but turned out to be true, I knew I would have to dig in. So I pored through the research, sifted through databases, and realized that the link in this case was too strong to dismiss.

It is a relationship that scientists have been looking at for years, and a counterintuitive one since thunderstorms are generally thought to clear the air of allergens. The bottom line is that almost every study that has examined the link has found overwhelming evidence to support it.

One of the most exhaustive studies, published in the journal *Thorax*, focused on the Atlanta area because the South has frequent thunderstorms and a high prevalence of asthma cases. Conducted by a team of climatologists and epidemiologists, the study involved looking at over 10 million emergency room visits in forty-one hospitals during an eleven-year period. After looking specifically at 215,832 asthma emergency room visits during that period, the team found that 28,350 occurred on days that followed thunderstorms, resulting in at least a 3 percent higher incidence compared to days that did not follow storms. That figure may not sound like much, but in a city of millions of people, it could translate to thousands of cases—and many needless deaths.

A number of other studies over the years, conducted in

countries from Canada to England to Australia, have also found spikes in the number of cases after stormy weather. The reason is something of a mystery, but three strong ones have been proposed, and it's possible that all three scenarios play a role. Thunderstorms may prompt the release of asthma-triggering starch particles, spread pollutants, and rupture pollen grains, making them small enough to enter the airways.

Do changes in the weather cause heart attacks?

Perhaps all those snowbirds who flee south for the winter are on to something. Instead of simply gaining warmer climates, it may also be better health that they're after, because as summer turns to autumn and the cold of winter hangs on the horizon, speculation that cold snaps spur heart attacks invariably arises.

It's a link that has been asserted—and not to mention disputed—for some time, and for all sorts of reasons. We know from medical observations that drops in temperature can lead to inflammation from common colds and influenza, higher blood pressure from narrowed blood vessels, and increased clotting caused by increasingly viscous blood. Even the stress and indulgence of the holiday season—squabbles with the in-laws, for instance, or nights of heavy feasting and one too many swigs from that bottle of Old Grandad—would seem to heighten the risk.

So it's small wonder that as scientists have finally turned to epidemiological studies to uncover a connection, they have found one.

One of the largest and most intriguing of these studies used data from the World Health Organization to look at changes in weather and heart attack rates in women that occurred over fifty years in seventeen countries on four continents. Overall, the authors found that a 5-degree drop in temperature was associated, in general, with a 7 percent increase in admissions for stroke, as well as a 12 percent rise in admissions for heart attack.

Another study by researchers in France looked at seven hundred hospital admissions over a two-year period. They found that in people with hypertension, the risk of suffering a heart attack doubled when the temperature fell below 25 degrees Fahrenheit (minus 4 degrees Celsius) and, in addition, that it climbed by 62 percent when there was a 5-degree difference between the day of the attack and the day preceding it.

To be sure, there has been at least one study that has argued otherwise. That one, by Canadian researchers, found no connection at all between heart attack rates and Chinook winds in Calgary—which can cause temperatures to swing wildly. But many more studies have indeed confirmed a link.

If you're like me, you might be thinking that an annual trip to Miami at the start of every winter may be in order. Beautiful people, balmy weather, *and* better protection against a heart attack! What exactly could go wrong? Well, before you book your tickets, keep in mind one thing: Florida and other warm environs experience increases in heart attacks during the winter season as well. So snowbirds are not entirely protected.

So what gives?

Two words: flu season. It coincides with winter, even in warm climates, and influenza can spur inflammation that taxes the heart. But all is not lost. Whether you plan to stick around or head south for the winter, just make sure you get your flu shot on schedule—it could very well ward off more than just a fever.

CAN MISTLETOE BE DEADLY? WHAT ABOUT POINSETTIAS?

That Christmas bough of mistletoe that you left around a little too long last year has a legendary reputation for romance, but it is also widely considered as lethal as it is festive. It's no wonder that every November and December, calls to poison control centers spike, and health authorities warn of the dangers of the plant, typically sending out "holiday safety" fliers warning people to keep mistletoe out of the reach of children and pets, lest there be fatal consequences.

Although many people consider every part of the plant toxic, it's the berries that are particularly dangerous. And in reality, studies show that mistletoe in general is not quite as hazardous as it is made out to be. The plant does in fact contain harmful chemicals, like viscotoxins, a group of small proteins that can cause gastrointestinal distress, a slowed heartbeat, and other unfortunate side effects. But ingesting mistletoe is a bit like sitting through a bad movie: it'll hurt, but it probably won't kill you. You run a greater risk of bodily harm by going shopping at a crowded Toys "R" Us on Christmas Eve.

In studies of hundreds of cases of accidental mistletoe ingestion over the years, there were no fatalities and only a handful of severe reactions. One study published in 1996 looked at ninety-two cases of mistletoe ingestion and found that only a small fraction of patients showed any symptoms. Eight of ten people who consumed five or more berries had no symptoms, and three of the eleven people who consumed only leaves had upset stomachs.

Other studies have found similar effects, suggesting that while mistletoe can be toxic, its lethal reputation is not quite deserved.

Then there is poinsettia, that radiant, red-topped shrub celebrated for its beauty and also feared for its rumored toxicity. Next to mistletoe, no other plant is more closely associated with the holidays. The plant, native to Mexico, was introduced in the United States in the 1820s by Joel Robert Poinsett, the first ambassador to Mexico. But it was only a century later, in 1919, that it gained a reputation for deadliness, when a two-year-old boy died in Hawaii and the cause was mistakenly attributed to poinsettia ingestion.

But like mistletoe, studies show that poinsettias can be problematic but not exactly deadly. Like many members of the plant genus Euphorbia, poinsettias have sap that can irritate the skin and cause an upset stomach if consumed in large enough quantities.

That appears to be about it. One study found that in rats, poinsettia was not toxic even at extremely high doses—luckily, for the rats. Another study, in the *American Journal of Emergency Medicine*, found not one fatality among 22,793 cases of poinsettia exposures reported to poison control centers nationwide. About 93 percent of the cases involved children. The majority of people exposed did not receive treatment at a medical center, and about 92 percent showed no signs of sickness at all.

In other words, it may be a good idea to keep poinsettias away from the curious paws and arms of pets and children, but no need to cross them off the holiday shopping list. Consider it one less thing to worry about when the holidays roll around. As for in-laws, the extra weight, and those inescapable TV reruns of *It's a Wonderful Life*—well, those will always be an unavoidable nuisance.

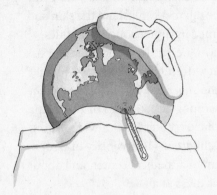

10
WORLD HEALTH

One Big Ball of Germs

The rest of the world needs love too!

Until recently, that concept had not fully dawned on me. But after the publication of *Never Shower in a Thunderstorm*, I began noticing a refrain in my conversations with people who were born or raised in other countries. I would hear, "You know, in my country, a lot of people believe . . ." or "My great grandmother and my other relatives back home always used to tell me that."

In my quest to squeeze the truth out of the old wives' tales and medical rumors we're all so accustomed to hearing, it seems that I left a few stones unturned. I had failed to plumb some of the more prevalent health and fitness beliefs circulating in other parts of the world, leaving them as neglected as a tourist in Paris asking for directions to "that Effin Tower thing."

Pretty soon, that omission became even more conspicuous

when it became clear how tightly intertwined American and foreign folklore can sometimes be. Many health sayings seem uniquely American because we grew up with them—we learn them from our parents, share them with our friends, and pass them down through generations. But in fact they have foreign ancestry. And that's especially true of the most popular ones.

The notion that eating carrots is good for your eyes, as we learned, was a bogus cover story concocted in England back in World War II, when the Royal Air Force came up with it to hide their use of radar, saying that British fighter pilots were shooting down enormous numbers of enemy aircraft simply because they ate lots of carrots. And the idea that chocolate can inspire feelings of lust and romance came to life in Mexico, where, I discovered, the emperor Montezuma considered it a sort of Viagra, and in France, where Madame du Barry, a mistress of Louis XV, insisted that all her lovers consume it before joining her for sexual trysts.

Those were claims that I examined in detail in *Never Shower in a Thunderstorm.* Now it's time to take a closer look at some claims that are prevalent in other countries but for whatever reason have not quite made the full leap to the United States—or at least not yet. So I set out on an odd mission, tracking down expatriate friends and acquaintances and quizzing them on the medical folklore most ingrained in their native cultures. Then I sifted through books, foreign publications, and the medical literature to verify the acceptance—and veracity—of the most intriguing claims.

They range from the wacky, like the one in Ireland about Guinness doing a body good, to the deadly serious, like the widespread concern in sub-Saharan Africa that bloodsucking mosquitoes can transmit HIV. And in some cases they are claims that have captured international headlines. You may recall hearing in the wake of the tsunami that struck southern Asia in 2004 that large contingents of animals fled to higher ground and safer areas long before humans had any inkling that a catastrophe was in the offing, apparently because some animals have a sort of sixth sense for natural disaster. An intriguing connection, but is it true?

Flip through to find out—no passport required.

CAN ANIMALS TELL WHEN A NATURAL DISASTER IS ABOUT TO STRIKE? DO THEY HAVE A SIXTH SENSE?

The tsunami that swept across the Indian Ocean in 2004, inflicting untold devastation and a death toll exceeding 200,000, baffled people around the globe. In its wake, some obvious questions followed: Why had no one predicted such a disastrous calamity, and how could it possibly have claimed so many lives? In the weeks and months that followed, as rescue workers sifted through what remained and uncovered the full extent of the devastation, people in the region took note of a strange phenomenon, and they asked another question: Where are all the dead animals?

The bodies of numerous tourists and locals who drowned in the surge of powerful waves quickly surfaced, but there were almost no animal carcasses to speak of, leading many locals to argue that the animals had sensed the disaster before it occurred.

To be sure, it is not as though the many wild and domesticated animals in the region were beyond the tsunami's long reach. Floodwaters raced at least as far as two miles inland, buffeting a number of wildlife refuges and reserves. At Yala National Park in Sri Lanka, for example, the tsunami's waves killed tourists and park workers and destroyed buildings. Only 30 of the 250 tourist vehicles that reportedly entered the park that day returned to base later on. But despite all the animals that lived in the park—leopards, deer, jackals, elephants—there were no reports of animal deaths at Yala in the days after the disaster. As one BBC article published shortly after the catastrophe explained: "Wildlife officials in Sri Lanka have reported that, despite the loss of human life in the Asian disaster, there have been no recorded animal deaths."

Others spoke of anecdotal reports of animals throughout the region fleeing to higher ground before the tsunami struck, and they pointed to longtime reports of dogs and other pets behaving erratically just before major earthquakes in other countries, especially in China and Japan. In one famous incident in 1975, officials in Haicheng, a large city in China, began evacuating residents just days before a 7.3-magnitude earthquake ferociously shook the city—an action that spared tens of thousands of lives. Many people reported their animals behaving strangely before the quake, and it's believed that these reports are at least in part what spurred officials to act.

One researcher I contacted, Rupert Sheldrake, a biochemist who wrote the books *Dogs That Know When Their Owners Are Coming Home* and *The Sense of Being Stared At*, argued that many similar examples exist. Large numbers of people reported wild and domesticated animals suddenly showing signs of anxiety or unusual behavior before earthquakes in the city of Kobe in Japan in 1995, in Italy in 1997, and in Turkey in 1999. In that last case, Sheldrake said that people noticed their cats acting weirdly and their dogs howling for hours on end shortly before the quake jolted the country.

It would seem from all of this that animals have a sixth sense that allows them to sniff out oncoming disasters and escape or warn of them.

But there is a more realistic explanation. Scientists in China and Japan have studied the phenomenon for years, as have researchers at the United States Geological Survey. Their conclusion is that animals that behave strangely just before a major event like an earthquake or tsunami—events that are caused by mass movements and tectonic activity—can sense the subtle, low-frequency waves that are the first to shoot through the ground. Most humans are unable to detect these initial waves, known as P waves, and only notice the larger S waves that arrive afterward.

There are other precursors to significant quakes and events that occur hours or days beforehand and that some animals can detect, like ground tilting, groundwater changes, and electrical or magnetic field alterations. But research on these earlier indicators is limited. Animals that sense these changes—particularly the small P waves—may find them unnerving or a sign of impending danger and react instinctively by barking, behaving anxiously, or fleeing.

Elephants, for example, are known to use their trunks and feet—which are highly sensitive—to detect and interpret low-frequency seismic signals from other elephants. It's easy to see how they would have sensed disturbing seismic activity long before humans in Southeast Asia became aware of the tsunami. In fact, people in Thailand reported that elephants there became agitated and moved to higher ground shortly before the area was flooded.

Researchers believe that elephants may even have the ability to sense severe weather systems. "Elephants may be able to sense the environment better than we realize," Caitlin O'Connell-Rodwell, an ecologist who studies elephants, told the *Stanford Report*. "When it rains in Angola, elephants one hundred miles away in Etosha National Park start to move north in search of water. It could be that they are sensing underground vibrations generated by thunder."

Perhaps dogs, cats, and other sensitive animals are able to detect these environmental precursors as well.

But studies of whether animals can sense impending disaster have also revealed something else: many of the anecdotal reports about animal behavior are exaggerated. Remember those reports of no animal deaths at Yala National Park in Sri Lanka? A study that was published about a year and a half after the tsunami struck showed those early reports to be untrue. More than a dozen animal carcasses were recovered, including water buffalo, herons, a spotted deer, and peacocks. But no elephants, of course.

And remember that earthquake in Haicheng that Chinese officials predicted days in advance? Many scientists say it wasn't animal behavior that tipped them off, but a series of small tremors, called foreshocks, that raised concerns. That small detail was apparently left out of many media reports about the quake. Scientists, it seems, are just not as interesting as cats and dogs.

DOES EARLY TO BED, EARLY TO RISE, MAKE A MAN HEALTHY, WEALTHY, AND WISE?

There is no shortage of proverbs extolling the virtues of getting an early start to the day. Why stay in bed and let the day slip away when, we are told, the early bird gets the worm, those who lose an hour in the morning spend all day hunting for it, and, perhaps most inspiring of all, being early to bed and early to rise makes a man healthy, wealthy, and wise.

That last saying has long been attributed to Benjamin Franklin, Revolutionary War hero, signatory to the Declaration of Independence, and multitalented inventor who made such diverse contributions to society as the lightning rod, bifocal lenses, and a type of fireplace known as the Franklin stove. He also gave us numerous volumes of a wildly popular almanac—called *Poor Richard's Almanack*—that dispensed tidbits of knowledge and wise old adages like "There are no gains without pains," "Diligence is the mother of good luck," "Half the truth is often a great lie," and, of course, the aphorism at hand.

No doubt he was a great American. So it is easy to accept that if Benjamin Franklin decreed it, then there must be truth in it. Who would dare question the wisdom of a legendary founding father?

Well, humble as I usually strive to be, on this challenge, I'll bite. The gauntlet has been thrown. I submit that this saying is not an American one that our colonial forefathers coined, but a British one, decreed hundreds of years before it appeared in an American text. And more important, after a little digging, and a quick perusal of the medical literature, I must question the proverb's underlying veracity.

First, according to historians with unusual knowledge of the origins of certain proverbs, the saying seems to have first appeared in the English language in 1496, when a variation was included in *A Treatyse of Fysshynge wyth an Angle*, which was written by Dame Juliana Berners and is considered the earliest known book on sport fishing. Berners was a nun who lived in the south of England—in Hertfordshire, to be exact—and though her words are a bit difficult to decipher on first glance, a close look at one of her passages is revealing:

> Also who soo woll vse the game of anglynge: *he must ryse erly*. Whiche thyng is prouffrable to man in this wyse / That is to wyte: moost to the heele of his soule. For it shall cause hym to be hole. *Also to the encrease of his goodys. For it shall make hym ryche. As the olde englysshe prouverbe sayth in this wyse. Who soo woll ryse erly shall be holy helthy & zely.* (Italics added).

While the phrases in this passage are not identical to the proverb familiar to us today, it's clear that this is an early version of it, which over time evolved into the saying that was published in *Poor Richard's Almanack*. Dame Berners also points out that her advice stems from an "olde englysshe prouverbe," suggesting that saying dates back even further.

But the more important question, it would seem, is whether

those who make a habit of rising early and going to sleep early tend to be better off than night owls like me, who prefer to stay up late and sleep in a little longer.

Appropriately enough, the very scientists who first put this maxim to the test hail from Southampton University, located in Hampshire County in the south of England, not far from the home of Dame Berners. In their study, funded by the Department of Health and Social Security, the team from Southampton tracked the health, wealth, and sleeping habits of more than 1,229 men and women across England over more than two decades. They found that people who rise and fall asleep early—called larks—were no richer or healthier than the night owls who slept in late. Nor did they show better cognitive performance. Overall, in fact, the owls tended to have the largest mean income.

Those results gibe with the findings of a later study by researchers at Harvard University and the Beth Israel Deaconess Medical Center in Boston. The scientists looked at 950 adults and found that the mortality of early-to-bed, early-to-risers did not differ significantly from that of other groups. They also found no relationship among sleep habits, wealth, and educational attainment.

Apparently, it's not what time you *start* your day, but what you ultimately *do* with it that matters.

But the earlier, British study did find one concerning finding: people who averaged twelve or more hours of sleep each night had a far higher risk of early death than those who slept nine hours or less. They were one and a half times more likely to die during the study. The authors were not sure why that was the case. But most scientists don't think there is anything fundamentally dangerous about excessive sleep. It's more likely that people who sleep that much may have an undiagnosed, underlying illness that causes fatigue and earlier death.

If you find yourself regularly needing twelve or more hours of sleep each night, better get yourself to a doctor for a checkup.

And now that we know getting up early won't necessarily do you any good, feel free to make it an afternoon appointment.

CAN HONEY SOOTHE A COUGH AND OTHER RESPIRATORY AILMENTS?

Growing up in a household run by two parents who were perhaps the most health-conscious people I've ever known—my mother, a vegan, at times even shunned medicine, preferring to deliver six of her seven children naturally, without morphine—I became a sucker for natural cures. Of course, as I got older and fell in love with science, I questioned every health claim I heard until I could find a study to verify it. But still, I always believed, and still do to this day, that drugs are not the answer to every medical ailment, and alternative medicine does have some bright spots.

So when I started hearing over and over again from people with Middle Eastern upbringings that an old-time cure for colds and other respiratory conditions from their part of the world was plain and simple honey, my curiosity was stoked. The reporter in me raised a skeptical eyebrow, but the little boy who struggled with asthma for years wanted the details.

It turns out that honey has been considered medicine in Islamic culture for ages, going all the way back to the Qur'an, which touted honey as a balm for various health conditions. "And thy Lord taught the bee to build its cells in hills, on trees and in habitations," one passage states. "There issues from within their bodies a drink of varying colors, wherein is healing for mankind. Verily in this is a Sign for those who give thought."

There is plenty of research in more modern texts outlining the antioxidants and other healthy compounds found in honey. But it's only recently that studies have examined whether this ancient claim has any merits. So far, the evidence is tantalizing.

In 2008, scientists showed that honey may be effective against chronic rhinosinusitis, which can be extremely hard to treat. Specifically, they showed that honey helps eliminate biofilms, the complex aggregates of microorganisms that appear to be behind many cases of antibiotic-resistant forms of the condition. It's estimated that as many as 80 percent of people who undergo surgery for chronic rhinosinusitis may have these biofilms in their sinus cavities.

On a related matter, another study, this one published in the *Archives of Pediatric and Adolescent Medicine*, found that a spoonful of honey could eliminate a child's cough more safely and effectively than conventional cough medicines. In the study, scientists recruited a group of 105 children, ages two to eighteen, who had upper-respiratory infections and randomly assigned each subject to one of three groups: one that received no treatment, a second that received one or two teaspoons of honey, and a third that received honey-flavored dextromethorphan. They found that the honey worked like a charm (though because of the risk of infant botulism, honey should never be given to children under one year of age unless it has been certified as free of spores).

For the record, the study was funded at least in part by the National Honey Board, "an industry-backed agency of the Department of Agriculture." More evidence is needed, but overall, based on the aforementioned studies and others, there's good reason to think that when it comes to some common upper-respiratory conditions, a little bit of honey may do some good.

CAN POMEGRANATES INCREASE VIRILITY?

In China, when something momentous occurs and friends and family want to offer their congratulations, they do so by handing out pomegranates.

The delicious red fruit, with its many seeds—its name literally meaning "seeded apple" in Latin—symbolizes fertility in China. The fruit can often be found in traditional Chinese paintings, representing good luck, fortune, and fertility. Giving someone a pomegranate implies that the person will have lots of children. As a friend from China once explained to me, pomegranate juice is considered the vegetable Viagra.

In a country that experienced such an incredible explosion in population that a one-child policy was instituted in 1979, the centuries-long obsession with the pomegranate may help to explain things. As a report in the *British Medical Journal* pointed out in 2000, "In China the pomegranate is widely represented in ceramic art symbolizing fertility, abundance, posterity, numerous and virtuous offspring, and a blessed future. A picture of a ripe open pomegranate is a popular wedding present."

Symbolism can have powerful effects on the human psyche. But studies of what pomegranate can do for fertility have so far offered a limited endorsement. In 2008, for example, researchers found that regular consumption of pomegranate juice could protect against damage to the fatty acids in sperm, apparently because of the juice's high antioxidant content. The study found that the juice also provided "an increase in epididymal sperm concentration, sperm motility, spermatogenic cell density and . . . it decreased abnormal sperm rate when compared to the control group."

The problem? It was a laboratory study on animals, which suggests some promise, but is not considered solid evidence since animal studies are often only preliminary. Other scientists have found evidence that pomegranate juice can reduce blood pressure and improve blood flow, problems that can contribute to erectile dysfunction. And while we're down in that region, compounds in pomegranate have been shown to play at least a small role in reducing the risk of prostate cancer.

But the evidence for virility, at best, is what I like to call circumstantial. Good, but not good enough.

ARE THOSE AÇAI BERRY DRINKS
ALL THEY'RE CRACKED UP TO BE?

Fad health foods are about as abundant these days as flies at a butcher shop. Remember the grapefruit craze of the 1980s and '90s, when throngs of people insisted it was a good idea to load up on grapefruit to lose weight? Or the claim that gorging on cabbage soup could improve health and help you shed pounds? Or what about the yogurt fad of the '90s, based on the belief that yogurt could extend your life span because all those centenarians in the Caucasus Mountains swore by it?

We know now that loading up on grapefruit and cabbages to the exclusion of other healthful foods is obviously a bad idea. And it turns out that the supposedly high concentration of yogurt-eating centenarians in the Caucasus Mountains was doubtful, since very few of those claiming to be in their hundreds were able to produce verifiable birth records.

These fad health foods come and go with such regularity that it's easy to barely even give some of them a second look. But it's hard not to pay attention to the latest super food that's sweeping the globe, the açai berry, that large blueberry-like fruit that's harvested deep in the Brazilian rain forest from açai palms. Long a secret of the Amazon, and prized for its supposed medicinal properties throughout Brazil, the açai berry has exploded in popularity in recent years. Sales of açai berries have soared in the United States and other countries, and it's almost impossible to walk into a grocery store or supermarket without seeing açai-based beverages on the shelves. Sales of açai products in the United States alone climbed to $13.5 million in 2007, up from $435,000 two years previously, according to Spins Inc., a natural-food tracker. Part of that may have been fueled by the fact that açai products were featured on *Oprah* and the *Rachael Ray Show*.

But they're expensive. Some bottles of the stuff go for as much as forty bucks a pop.

And it's no wonder. Açai berries have been credited with all sorts of amazing health benefits. It's said they can boost metabolism, increase energy, ease arthritis, melt away pounds, reverse wrinkles, improve cardiovascular health, and lower cholesterol. And I'm pretty sure I've heard they can do your taxes, too.

All of this has been attributed to antioxidants. The buzz about açai berries is that, pound for pound, they contain far more antioxidants than any other fruit or vegetable. Antioxidants can do some pretty remarkable things. They're the compounds that give red wine and green tea their amazing health benefits, and studies have suggested that a diet high in antioxidants might reduce the risk of a number of diseases. They're even used as medication to treat certain types of brain injury. In other words, you definitely want a lot of antioxidants in your diet.

But don't believe the companies touting açai berries as the best source of antioxidants. A good source, sure, but you can find better sources for less. One 2006 study that looked at the antioxidant content of various fruits found that açai came in fifth, behind mangoes and grapes. At the top of the list was acerola, also known as the Barbados cherry or wild crape myrtle, which is found in Texas, Mexico, Brazil and other parts of South America, and the Caribbean.

Another study found that açai seems to have a mild inhibitory effect on COX-1 and COX-2, which are enzymes in the body that seem to promote pain. Suppressing the COX enzymes reduces pain and inflammation, which is how nonsteroidal anti-inflammatory drugs, or NSAID, like aspirin and ibuprofen, operate. Vioxx, the popular painkiller, is a COX-2 inhibitor, although it was pulled off the market in 2004 because it was found to increase the risk of heart attack and stroke.

In any case, the mild COX-inhibiting effects of açai may explain why some arthritis patients feel it eases their symptoms. As of 2008, however, there hasn't been any scientific evidence proving that açai berries work any better than prescription drugs and over-the-counter medications. A third study found that antioxidant compounds in açai could destroy leukemia cancer cells—but that was only seen in test tubes, which is not exactly groundbreaking.

In fact, of all the studies that have examined the health benefits of açai berries, none have shown that regularly consuming açai products is superior to regularly consuming other high-antioxidant fruits—or even that doing so lowers your risk of the aforementioned diseases at all. No one is saying it doesn't, but unless you've got money to burn, there's no solid scientific evidence that should propel you to pay a premium for açai products when you can probably get as much benefit from heading down to your local grocer and picking up a bag of grapes, a few mangoes, and some blueberries, which are also high in antioxidants.

In other words, save your money.

Is Guinness good for your health?

In the United States, drinking to good health means a glass of wine. It's impossible to read anything that discusses alcohol and health (including this book) without being reminded of all the benefits that come from uncorking a good bottle of red or white.

But beer lovers rejoice! In Ireland there's an entirely different saying: "Guinness Is Good for You." Or as my friends back in Dublin never ceased to remind me as we sipped pints of the dark brew at the local pubs, "A Guinness a day keeps the doctor away."

This by no means is to be taken lightly.

Guinness dates at least back to the 1700s, and the medical benefits ascribed to it probably go that far back as well. But the notion of Guinness as medicine became official in the 1920s, when its maker discovered in surveys of the Irish public that the thing people liked about it above anything else was most intangible. Put simply, they responded, it made them feel good. Pretty soon, the "Guinness Is Good for You" slogan was slapped on labels, and people were toasting to good health, pints in hand.

Small children and nursing mothers were encouraged to imbibe small amounts of the drink because of its high iron content. Men were counting on it as an aphrodisiac. And patients throughout the United Kingdom were being served Guinness in hospitals to help them recover from surgery.

The slogan eventually fell out of favor and is no longer seen in ads or on labels, but the belief persists—for good reason. And I'm not just saying that because my last name is O'Connor.

For starters, plenty of studies have found that beer has the same health benefits as wine. That is, at least, when it's consumed in moderation, as in no more than two servings a day. For example, one study in the *New England Journal of Medicine* found that light to moderate beer drinkers reduce their odds of suffering a stroke by 20 percent—a benefit that could be seen with as little as one drink a week. Other studies have found that it decreases coronary artery disease by 30 percent, increases levels of B vitamins in the blood, relaxes blood vessels, and raises HDL cholesterol, the good kind.

But that's just beer in general. Darker beers tend to have more healthful compounds, and Guinness in particular is loaded with them. A study by researchers at the University of Wisconsin in 2004 found that the drink is packed with a class of antioxidants known as flavonoids, the same compounds that give many dark fruits and vegetables their color, and which prevent LDL cholesterol—the bad kind—from gumming up blood vessels. In the study, a serving of Guinness worked even better than lagers like Heineken, a lighter beer, at preventing the type of blood clots that can set off heart attacks.

Need any more reason to grab a pint? Yeah, didn't think so.

Next time you're in Ireland, you can find a good place to grab one with a simple question, which any local can answer: "Where can I find good crack?" That's not something you'd ever ask in the United States. But in Dublin, crack, sometimes spelled *craic*, refers to fun, enjoyment, and hearty drinking. You'll want a place, in other words, that has good people, music, dancing, and crack. Of course in Ireland, that's never hard to find.

CAN EATING LICORICE RAISE YOUR BLOOD PRESSURE?

From its arid deserts in the north to its verdant landscape in the south, the continent of Africa is speckled with communities and cultures that consider the licorice root a staple.

Since ancient times, it's been used as a potent spice in dishes, but it has also found a medicinal life. Licorice root, referred to in Africa as "chew sticks," is still widely used as an expectorant, an ingredient in cough syrups, a balm of sorts for ulcers, and a mild laxative. But walk the streets of African communities in cities like New York, where licorice root is sold by the bucketful in African groceries, and it's clear that one of the more popular reasons it's promoted is for its effects on blood pressure.

Licorice, an old African saying goes, can cure low blood pressure, a condition that can indicate good health in some people—particularly athletes—but a serious problem for others, particularly the elderly. It can set off poor blood flow to vital organs like the brain, heart, and lungs.

Many natural plants and herbs touted as miracle remedies fail to meet muster, but don't count licorice in that category.

The active substance in licorice is glycyrrhetinic acid, a compound with a mouthful-of-a-moniker that gives the root its curiously strong but slow-acting sweet flavor. Besides being more than thirty times as potent as sucrose, or table sugar, glycyrrhetinic acid has been shown in recent studies to have a profound effect on blood pressure. It's not known why or by what mechanism the compound accomplishes this—it's believed it may force the body to retain sodium and expel potassium—but studies have shown that regular consumption of even small amounts of licorice root can cause blood pressure to spike dramatically in a matter of days or weeks.

In a study in the *Journal of Human Hypertension*, scientists found that subjects who chewed a moderate amount of licorice in one sitting saw their levels of systolic blood pressure (the top number in a blood pressure reading) jump by 3.1 to 14.4 points. And after two weeks of chewing a small amount daily—about 50 grams, or roughly 1.8 ounces—the subjects experienced "a significant rise in blood pressure," the authors found.

That can be helpful for some hypotensive people who can use a boost in their readings, but it can be dangerous for people with normal to high blood pressure. And it can cause other side effects, like low potassium and liver damage. One fifty-six-year-old woman in England gained notoriety in 2004 when she showed up at a hospital with muscle problems, low potassium, and high blood pressure. The diagnosis: too much licorice. She had a habit of eating a packet a day.

You might want to have a good idea of where your blood pressure stands before you indulge in licorice. But in the United States and many other countries, keep in mind that it's usually only the imported varieties of licorice that have these side effects. The red stuff we know as Twizzlers and by other names is not real licorice, and many licorice-flavored lozenges and candies contain artificial flavors, not real licorice extract. The only way to know for sure is to look at the list of ingredients.

CAN HIV BE TRANSMITTED THROUGH MOSQUITOES?

It seems like common sense.

If a bloodsucking mosquito bites a person infected with a disease, then the next person attacked by that mosquito should be at risk of becoming infected when the pest injects its saliva into the unfortunate and unsuspecting host. This is how yellow fever, the West Nile virus, some types of encephalitis, and of course malaria are spread among people. So shouldn't that apply to HIV as well?

In sub-Saharan Africa—a region that has a mere 10 percent of the world's population but more than 60 percent of all people living with HIV—this belief is particularly widespread. Many doctors and AIDS consultants in southern Africa say they are sometimes inundated with questions about the link, and that it cuts across people of every background, race, and class: whites, blacks, the poor, even the educated.

While it may sound feasible, solid studies have proven that it isn't possible. One of the first agencies to investigate the theory was the Centers for Disease Control and Prevention, which delved into it because the concerns were so widespread and the ramifications frightening. Mosquitoes may be insufferable pests who torture humans in many ways, but for a number of reasons they are unable to infect their hosts with HIV.

For starters, mosquitoes do not inject blood into a person when they bite—only saliva, which acts as a lubricant to help them feed more easily. Malaria and other diseases that are well established as mosquito-borne can be transmitted through saliva, but HIV, on the other hand, cannot. According to the CDC, the virus lives for only a short time in mosquitoes and insects, before quickly dying without reproducing.

Even if a mosquito did bite a person infected with HIV, it

wouldn't transfer it to another person because mosquitoes do not jump from one person to the next. Instead, they extract their bloody meal and then retreat to a safe place to digest it, before finding their next human dinner. They are also not known to be messy eaters: their mouths don't usually end up covered in blood, so there's little chance of any being transferred from their mouth to a person's body.

If that all sounds theoretical and uncertain, it's not. Intense epidemiological studies by the CDC and other agencies have found no evidence of HIV transmission through insects even in areas of southern Africa where HIV is common and mosquitoes are ubiquitous. If the disease were transmitted that easily by pests, then far more seniors would be infected, experts say. Instead, the majority of cases are among sexually active populations and children who were infected at birth.

WHY WAS THERE AN EXPLOSION IN MALE BABIES IN POSTWAR EUROPE?

In the aftermaths of World Wars I and II, scientists noticed an unusual phenomenon in countries throughout Europe, particularly in countries along the Mediterranean, from Portugal to Italy to Bulgaria. There were the usual explosions in babies across the continent, as is typically expected after a long and costly war, when men return, couples reunite, and the business of baby making experiences a resurgence.

But in many European countries, the ratio of male to female babies took an unexpected turn. Suddenly there was a sharp increase in the proportion of male babies being born, which continued for several years after each war. In some European countries after World War I, for example, an extra two boys were born for every one hundred girls.

All sorts of theories were proposed. Perhaps only the largest, strongest soldiers had returned from the war, and were more likely to father male babies. Or perhaps the returning soldiers were having lots and lots of sex, and somehow impregnating their significant others during the time in their cycles when they are more likely to have male babies. No one knew for sure, and it remained a mystery for some time.

But in recent years, a solid explanation sprang forth. And it answered another simmering question: Are some men more likely to father boys? That second question stems from anecdotal observations that men who come from families with plenty of males seem to have higher odds of fathering boys, and that for men with many sisters, it's vice versa.

Well, that observation was no illusion: it's true. And what seems to happen is that during major wars, men who are more likely to father boys gain a brief advantage.

We know this because in 2008, an insightful study published in the journal *Evolutionary Biology* examined the histories of more than nine hundred American and European families dating to 1600, involving more than half a million people. A child's sex is always determined by the father, since men cast the deciding chromosome—either an X or a Y—whereas women produce eggs that carry an X chromosome. The study produced evidence that men carry a gene that determines the percentage of X and Y chromosomes in their sperm, and that the gene comes in three alleles, or versions. One produces mostly X chromosomes, another mostly Y, and the third yields equal numbers of both.

Now let's look at what happens during a world war. Let's look at two different men, one who carries the gene that leads to more boys, and another who carries the gene for more girls. Let's say each man has four adult children. The first male sires three sons and one daughter. The second man fathers three daughters and one son. Let's say each man's sons—who are all adults—go off to fight in the war. It's obvious that first father—who has more boys—has greater odds of seeing a son return from war, because even if two of his boys are killed in action, the third one might survive. Think of the movie *Saving Private Ryan*. The second father, meanwhile—who passed his "girl" gene on to his son—has only one boy, and has lower odds of seeing that one boy return.

Now, broaden this out on a much larger scale, and you see that there should be a greater proportion of men with the "boy" gene returning from war and, subsequently, producing babies.

But after a while, things even out again. When the proportion of males in the population surges, women are likely to have a much easier time finding a mate, so men who had all those daughters will suddenly see their genes come back again.

Of course, keep in mind that carrying a gene that predisposes men to more sons or daughters is no guarantee, in the way that rolling a rigged die with a six on four of its faces and a three on the other two is no guarantee of landing a six every time. But it does mean that with enough rolls of the die, there will almost certainly be a higher number of sixes. Or, in this case, boys.

CAN HOT PEPPERS CURE AN ULCER?

Only in India, the land of spice, would the answer to a stomach ulcer be heat.

In the United States, it has long been suspected that spicy foods—along with stress, alcohol, and other harsh or acidic foods—cause ulcers. Eventually it was discovered that in reality, about 80 percent of all stomach ulcers are caused by a type of bacteria, called *H. pylori*. But the link between spice and ulcers—as a cause of them, or an aggravator—persists. Try serving Tabasco sauce to someone with an ulcer. You'd have an easier time getting your dog to eat cabbage.

And yet in India, chili peppers have long been used to treat a range of gastrointestinal conditions, from indigestion and mild discomfort to stomach ulcers. If it sounds like dumping accelerant on a forest fire, it's not. The people of India are on to something, which might explain why these uses for capsaicin, the active ingredient in cayenne pepper, have stuck around so long. Studies suggest that not only is capsaicin *not* an irritant to ulcers, it can actually relieve them.

I haven't seen anything this hot and healthy since Jane Fonda.

Other than *H. pylori*, one of the more common causes of ulcers is aspirin, which can cause damage to the mucosal membrane that lines the stomach. But when scientists had people regularly use aspirin over the course of about four weeks, they found that taking a small amount of capsaicin just before swallowing the aspirin had a protective effect. Endoscopies showed that the people who consumed capsaicin with their aspirin only scored on average about a 1.5 on a scale of "gastric injury," compared to an average of 4 among the people who did not take the capsaicin.

That kind of effect is clear outside in the real world too—beyond the confines of a controlled study. Epidemiological studies in Singapore, for example, have found that gastric ulcers are three times more common among the Chinese than among their Indian and Malaysian counterparts, who consume far more capsaicin. It seems that the idea most people have of capsaicin, the idea that it creates a harsh, acidic environment in the stomach that burns at the gastric lining much like capsaicin burns the eyes and fingertips, is wrong. One study put it this way: "Capsaicin does not stimulate but inhibits acid secretion, stimulates alkali, mucus secretions and particularly gastric mucosal blood flow, which help in prevention and healing of ulcers. Capsaicin acts by stimulating afferent neurons in the stomach and signals for protection against injury-causing agents."

That means if you're concerned about ulcers, you won't do

yourself any favors by avoiding foods with a little kick from capsaicin. You're better off digging in.

Besides, while you're munching away on that spicy Indian dish, you can chew on this, too: epidemiological research shows that people in Asia who regularly consume spicy curry dishes have a much lower risk of dementia and Alzheimer's disease than those who don't.

It seems that turmeric, one of the main ingredients in curry, has potent antioxidant and anti-inflammatory powers that help protect the brain from the plaques and tangles seen in Alzheimer's.

Good for the gut, good for the brain. That's not a bad combination.

EPILOGUE

Exercising the Brain

And here we find ourselves, at the end of another journey. But I hate good-byes, and before those curtains hit the stage floor, there is still time for one more twist.

Wrapping up a science book is always a good time to go over and consolidate all the facts worth remembering—facts that can come in handy over dinner, at a bar, or simply when you need to tell a parent, "I told you so." It's a habit I find myself increasingly engaging in, what with my rapidly dwindling reserves of brain power. But you may have heard, as I've often been told, that with the right exercises, you can train your brain to function at a higher level. Like bench presses for the mind, these training exercises are supposed to strengthen your brain, improving your intelligence and even preventing the mental decline that can precede Alzheimer's disease.

Certainly, there is a sizable population of people who would desperately want to know. In 2009, Americans are expected to spend $80 million on brain exercise products—forty times what was spent in 2005. Most of these products are computer programs that put you through challenging tasks that emphasize memory, quick reflexes, organization, and your ability to track moving objects. It's sort of like playing a video game, except without all the cool graphics, characters, or fun. Some exceptions do exist; for instance, games like Sudoku. To hear the companies who sell the more expensive products tell it—"Enhance your mental agility!" or "Your grandkids will thank you!"—you would have to be nuts not to drop a few hundred bucks for a whole library of them. But studies show that they may not be worth the moulah. It's not that you can't train your brain to increase its output. It's that there are much better options,

The problem with brain training programs is that it's not clear that the skills you gain when you excel at them apply to anything beyond those specific tasks. It seems that unless they challenge a broad range of skills, they have no real impact on general mental fitness. In one study, published in the *Journal of the American Medical Association* in 2002, for example, scientists recruited nearly three thousand older adults and split them into various groups, having each train with programs that emphasized either verbal memory, problem solving, or speed of processing. There was also one control group that received no training. At the end of the study, the subjects had improved at the individual tasks in which they had trained, but there was no evidence that their training had any impact on brain function outside of the context of those specific tasks—in other words, the training didn't appear to improve their everyday mental function.

Other studies have found that mental activities that are particularly challenging or stimulating—like studying art, learning a new language, or doing crossword puzzles—can help prevent a decline of mental faculties. They can keep the cobwebs from gathering under your skull. But they don't seem to have the ability to actually improve your cognitive abilities so much as *maintain* them.

But don't despair. There is one form of exercise that has been shown without a doubt to boost brain function: the physical kind. Odd, perhaps, but scientists have shown that physical exercise improves blood flow to the brain, stimulates the release of proteins that help form connections between brain cells, and boosts the number of brain cells in a part of the brain called the hippocampus, that forms and consolidates new memories. Physical fitness also seems to halt the natural shrinkage of the part of the brain that helps separate us from most other mammals, the frontal cortex, which is where our most sophisticated thought takes place.

So what does all this add up to? It means improvements in a variety of skills that fall under the umbrella term "executive function." That includes abilities like planning, problem solving, abstract thinking, and what's known as your "working memory." This type of memory acts something like the brain's notepad, helping you hold a telephone number in your head as you search for your Blackberry so you can type it in, for instance. Working memory generally fades as you age, which explains why you start to forget little things like where you put those car keys or why your parents can't remember what you just told them five minutes ago. The other executive function skills typically degrade as well.

Yet people who regularly engage in physical exercise don't show the same declines as their sedentary peers. Initially it was thought that people who are mentally sturdier are simply more likely to be active. But then it was discovered that when sedentary people become more physically active, it's not just their waistlines that benefit: their executive function shows signs of improvement as well.

A few other surprising habits that can help boost your brain power:

• Eat chocolate. An imaging study by scientists at the Nottingham medical school found that the antioxidants in cocoa "can increase the cerebral blood flow to gray matter," improving brain function. Pick dark chocolate over milk, since it has more antioxidants.

• Watch your posture. Studies have found that poor posture puts strain on your spine and compresses arteries, decreasing blood flow to the brain. Maybe that's why I feel like taking a nap every time I hunch over my desk.

• Get enough sleep. It helps you retain knowledge by consolidating memories and information you gathered during the day.

• Watch your diet. High amounts of unhealthy fats—the trans and saturated kinds—not only add inches to your waist, they can clog arteries and trigger brain-damaging strokes. Eat Omega-3s instead. They make up the outer membranes of brain cells, and studies suggest a high intake of Omega-3s improves brain function.

• Be alert for signs of depression. Scientists have found that depression reduces brain activity and can lead to patterns of brain function that resemble dementia.

But perhaps most important, now that the show is over, you should put down this book, get up, and get active. What's good for your body is good for your brain.

A Note to the Reader

This book may be a done deal, but the "Really?" column lives on, continuing to quash and confirm bizarre health claims every Tuesday in Science Times. If you've been following the column since before *Always Follow the Elephants* and *Never Shower in a Thunderstorm* hit stores, then you'll know, among other things, if taking the Pill (yes, that pill) can make you gain as much weight as everyone says it will, and whether drinking flat soda can *really* ease an upset stomach. Got a nagging health question that's been plaguing you that you'd love to get answered? Then put it to the test. E-mail me at scitimes@nytimes.com.

Notes

1. Kitchen First Aid

Introduction: B. S. Gold, R. C. Dart, and R. A. Barish, "Bites of Venomous Snakes," Review, *New England Journal of Medicine*, 347(5) (Aug. 1, 2002): 347–56. P. K. Visscher, R. S. Vetter, and S. Camazine, "Removing Bee Stings," *Lancet*, 348(9023) (Aug. 3, 1996): 301–2. A. O'Connor, "Really?" *New York Times*, Aug. 1, 2006.

Can a glass of warm milk cure insomnia?: J. Preuss (ed.), *Biblical and Talmudic Medicine* (Northvale, N.J.: Jason Aronson, 1993). "Effects of Normal Meals Rich in Carbohydrates or Proteins on Plasma Tryptophan and Tyrosine Ratios," *American Journal of Clinical Nutrition*, 77(1) (Jan. 2003): 128–32.

Can eating ginger cure motion sickness?: D. B. Mowrey and D. E. Clayson, "Motion Sickness, Ginger, and Psychophysics," *Lancet*, 1(8273) (Mar. 20, 1982): 655–57. A. Grøntved et al., "Ginger Root Against Seasickness: A Controlled Trial on the Open Sea," *Acta Oto-Laryngologica*, 105(1–2) (Jan.–Feb. 1988): 45–49.

Should you tilt your head back to treat a nosebleed?: The American Academy of Family Physicians, http://www.aafp.org/afp/20050115/305.html. J. A. Lavy and C. B. Koay, "First Aid Treatment of Epistaxis: Are the Patients Well Informed?" *Journal of Accident and Emergency Medicine*, 13(3) (May 1996): 193–95.

Can a pat of butter soothe a burn?: U.S. Centers for Disease Control and Prevention on treating burns/avoiding butter: http://www.bt.cdc.gov/masscasualties/burns.asp. P. C. Molan, "The Evidence Supporting the Use of Honey as a Wound Dressing," Review, *International Journal of Lower Extremity Wounds*, 5(1) (Mar. 2006): 40–54. Erratum in *International Journal of Lower Extremity Wounds*, 5(2) (June 2006): 122.

What about aloe vera gel?: R. Maenthaisong et al., "The Efficacy of Aloe Vera Used for Burn Wound Healing: A Systematic Review," *Burns*, 33(6) (Sept. 2007): 713–18. T. Kaufman et al., "Aloe Vera Gel Hindered Wound Healing of Experimental Second-Degree Burns: A Quantitative Controlled Study," *Journal of Burn Care Rehabilitation*, 9(2) (Mar.–Apr. 1988): 156–59. L. Cuttle et al., "The Efficacy of Aloe Vera, Tea Tree Oil and Saliva as First Aid Treatment for Partial Thickness Burn Injuries," *Burns*, 34:8 (July 4, 2008): 1176–82.

Can urine cure a jellyfish sting?: The "rapidly and completely" study is R. Hartwick, V. Callanan, and J. Williamson, "Disarming the Box-Jellyfish: Nematocyst Inhibition in *Chironex fleckeri*," *Medical Journal of Australia*, 1(1) (Jan. 12, 1980): 15–20. The shaving cream reference is in R. A. Perkins and S. S. Morgan, "Poisoning, Envenomation, and Trauma from Marine Creatures," *American Family Physician*, 69(4) (Feb. 15, 2004): 885–90.

Does CPR require mouth-to-mouth?: Holy Bible, Authorized King James Version, II Kings (4:32–37). SOS-KANTO Study Group, "Cardiopulmonary Resuscitation by Bystanders with Chest Compression Only (SOS-KANTO): An Observational Study," *Lancet*, 369(9565) (Mar. 17, 2007): 920–26. A. Hallstrom et al., "Cardiopulmonary Resuscitation by Chest Compression Alone or with Mouth-to-Mouth Ventilation," *New England Journal of Medicine*, 342(21) (May 25, 2000): 1546–53. That bystanders are more likely to intervene is discussed at http://emsresponder.com/print/EMS-Magazine/Cardiocerebral-Resuscitation/1$7857. The American Heart Association statement is at http://www.americanheart.org/presenter.jhtml?identifier=3057167.

Can super glue heal wounds?: A. J. Singer, J. V. Quinn, and J. E. Hollander, "The Cyanoacrylate Topical Skin Adhesives," Review, *American Journal of Emergency Medicine*, 26(4) (May 2008): 490–96. O. Karatepe et al., "To What Extent Is Cyanoacrylate Useful to Prevent Early Wound Infections in Hernia Surgery?" *Hernia*, 12(6) (June 5, 2008): 603–7.

Can chewing gum prevent heartburn?: R. Moazzez, D. Bartlett, and A. Anggiansah, "The Effect of Chewing Sugar-Free Gum on Gastroesophageal Reflux," *Journal of Dental Research*, 84(11) (Nov. 2005): 1062–65. B. Avidan et al., "Walking and Chewing Reduce Postprandial Acid Reflux," *Alimentary Pharmacology and Therapeutics*, 15(2) (Feb. 2001): 151–55.

Does breathing into a paper bag help you if you're hyperventilating?: M. Callaham, "Hypoxic Hazards of Traditional Paper Bag Rebreathing in Hyperventilating Patients," *Annals of Emergency Medicine*, 18(6) (June 1989): 622–28. M. A. Van den Hout et al., "Rebreathing to Cope with Hyperventilation: Experimental Tests of the Paper Bag Method," *Journal of Behavioral Medicine*, 11(3) (June 1988): 303–10.

Is hydrogen peroxide the best treatment for cuts and scrapes?: J. J. Leyden and N. M. Barelt, "Comparison of Topical Antibiotic Ointments, a Wound Protectant, and Antiseptics for the Treatment of Human Blister Wounds Contaminated with *Staphylococcus aureus*," *Journal of Family Practice*, 24(6) (June 1987): 601–4. W. Y. Lau and S. H. Wong, "Randomized, Prospective Trial of Topical Hydrogen Peroxide in Appendectomy Wound Infection: High Risk Factors," *American Journal of Surgery*, 142(3) (Sept. 1981): 393–97.

2. Regular Maintenance

Is it dangerous to swallow chewing gum?: D. E. Milov et al., "Chewing Gum Bezoars of the Gastrointestinal Tract," *Pediatrics*, 102(2) (Aug. 1998): e22. J. H. Truex, T. L. Silberman, and B. P. Wood, "Radiological Case of the Month: Bubble Gum Bezoar," *American Journal of Diseases of Children*, 143(2) (Feb. 1989): 253–54.

Are growing pains caused by growth spurts?: O. Friedland et al., "Decreased Bone Speed of Sound in Children with Growing Pains Measured by Quantitative Ultrasound," *Journal of Rheumatology*, 32(7) (July 2005): 1354–57. D. L. Picchietti and H. E. Stevens, "Early Manifestations of Restless Legs Syndrome in Childhood and Adolescence," *Sleep Medicine*, 9(7) (Oct. 2008): 770–81.

Can too much stress cause acne?: G. Yosipovitch et al., "Study of Psychological Stress, Sebum Production and Acne Vulgaris in Adolescents," *Acta Dermato-Venereologica*, 87(2) (Mar. 2007): 135–39.

Can vitamin E erase a scar?: M. Jenkins et al., "Failure of Topical Steroids and Vitamin E to Reduce Postoperative Scar Formation Following Reconstructive Surgery," *Journal of Burn Care Rehabilitation*, 7(4) (July–Aug. 1986): 309–12. The University of Miami study is L. S. Baumann and J. Spencer, "The Effects of Topical Vitamin E on the Cosmetic Appearance of Scars," *Dermatological Surgery*, 25(4) (Apr. 1999): 311–15.

Is drinking lots of water good for your skin?: R. C. Vreeman and A. E. Carroll, "Medical Myths," *British Medical Journal*, 335(7633) (Dec. 22, 2007): 1288–89. D. D. Wipke-Tevis and D. A. Williams, "Effect of Oral Hydration on Skin Microcirculation in Healthy Young and Midlife and Older Adults," *Wound Repair and Regeneration*, 15(2) (Mar.–Apr. 2007): 174–85. M. C. Cosgrove et al., "Dietary Nutrient Intakes and Skin-Aging Appearance Among Middle-Aged American Women," *American Journal of Clinical Nutrition*, 86(4) (Oct. 2007): 1225–31; erratum in *American Journal of Clinical Nutrition*, 88(2) (Aug. 2008): 480. L. B. Dunn et al., "Does Estrogen Prevent Skin Aging? Results from the First National Health and Nutrition Examination Survey (NHANES I)," *Archives of Dermatology*, 133(3) (Mar. 1997): 339–42.

Can smoking accelerate aging?: J. G. Mosley and A. C. Gibbs, "Premature Grey Hair and Hair Loss Among Smokers: A New Opportunity for Health Education?" *British Medical Journal*, 313(7072) (Dec. 21, 1996): 1616. L. H. Su and T. H. Chen, "Association of Androgenetic Alopecia with Smoking and Its Prevalence Among Asian Men: A Community-Based Survey," *Archives of Dermatology*, 143(11) (Nov. 2007): 1401–6. D. Model, "Smoker's Face: An Underrated Clinical Sign?" *British Medical Journal*, 291(6511) (Dec. 21–28, 1985): 1760–62. A. M. Valdes et al., "Obesity, Cigarette Smoking, and Telomere Length in Women," *Lancet*, 366(9486) (Aug. 20–26, 2005): 662–64.

Can acupuncture help you stop smoking?: A. Sood et al., "Complementary Treatments for Tobacco Cessation: A Survey," *Nicotine and Tobacco Research*, 8(6) (Dec. 2006): 767–71. A. R. White, H. Rampes, and J. L. Campbell, "Acupuncture and Related Interventions for Smoking Cessation," *Cochrane Database of Systematic Reviews*, 25(1) (Jan. 2006): CD000009. N. A. Christakis and J. H. Fowler, "The Collective Dynamics of Smoking in a Large Social Network," *New England Journal of Medicine*, 358(21) (May 22, 2008): 2249–58.

Are lefties more prone to migraines?: N. Geschwind and P. Behan, "Left-Handedness: Association with Immune Disease, Migraine, and Developmental Learning Disorder," *Proceedings of the National Academy of Sciences*, 79(16) (Aug. 1982): 5097–100. K. Biehl et al., "Migraine and Left-Handedness Are Not Associated: A New Case-Control Study and Meta-analysis," *Cephalalgia*, 28(5) (May 2008): 553–57. Published online Mar. 17, 2008.

Can cracking your neck cause a stroke?: K. P. Lee et al., "Neurologic Complications Following Chiropractic Manipulation: A Survey of California Neurologists," *Neurology*, 45(6) (June 1995): 1213–15. M. L. Miley et al., "Does Cervical Manipulative Therapy Cause Vertebral Artery Dissection and Stroke?" *Neurologist*, 14(1) (Jan. 2008): 66–73. J. D. Cassidy et al., "Risk of Vertebrobasilar Stroke and Chiropractic Care: Results of a Population-Based Case-Control and Case-Crossover Study," *Spine*, 33(4 Suppl.) (Feb. 15, 2008): S176–83. J. G. Heckmann et al., "Beauty Parlor Stroke Syndrome," *Cerebrovascular Diseases*, 21(1–2) (Jan. 2006): 140–41; published online May 28, 2004.

Can aspirin lower your risk of Alzheimer's disease?: M. Etminan, S. Gill, and A. Samii, "Effect of Non-steroidal Anti-inflammatory Drugs on Risk of Alzheimer's Disease: Systematic Review and Meta-analysis of Observational Studies," *British Medical Journal*, 327(7407) (July 19, 2003): 128. S. E. Nilsson et al., "Does Aspirin Protect Against Alzheimer's Dementia? A Study in a Swedish Population-Based Sample Aged > or = 80 Years," *European Journal of Clinical Pharmacology*, 59(4) (Aug. 2003): 313–19. K. M. Hayden et al., "Does NSAID Use Modify Cognitive Trajectories in the Elderly? The Cache County Study," *Neurology*, 69(3) (July 17, 2007): 275–82. J. H. Kang et al., "Low Dose Aspirin and Cognitive Function in the Women's Health Study Cognitive Cohort," *British Medical Journal*, 334(7601) (May 12, 2007): 987.

Is it dangerous to blow your nose when you have a cold?: J. M. Gwaltney Jr., J. O. Hendley, et al., "Nose Blowing Propels Nasal Fluid into the Paranasal Sinuses," *Clinical Infectious Diseases*, 30(2) (Feb. 2000): 387–91.

3. Calories Count

Is margarine healthier than butter?: F. B. Hu et al., "Dietary Fat Intake and the Risk of Coronary Heart Disease in Women," *New England Journal of Medicine*, 337(21) (Nov. 20, 1997): 1491–99.

Can grapefruit increase your risk of breast cancer?: K. R. Monroe et al., "Prospective Study of Grapefruit Intake and Risk of Breast Cancer in Postmenopausal Women: The Multiethnic Cohort Study," *British Journal of Cancer*, 97(3) (Aug. 6, 2007): 440–45. E. H. Kim et al., "A Prospective Study of Grapefruit and Grapefruit Juice Intake and Breast Cancer Risk," *British Journal of Cancer*, 98(1) (Jan. 15, 2008): 240–41.

Does mayonnaise make food spoil faster?: M. P. Doyle et al., "Fate of *Salmonella typhimurium* and *Staphylococcus aureus* in Meat Salads Prepared with Mayonnaise," *Journal of Food Protection*, 45 (Feb. 1982): 152–56. See also http://www.cdc.gov/ncidod/DBMD/diseaseinfo/files/foodborne_illness_FAQ.pdf.

Can too much cola cause kidney problems?: T. M. Saldana et al., "Carbonated Beverages and Chronic Kidney Disease," *Epidemiology*, 18(4) (July 2007): 501–6. Reported at http://abcnews.go.com/GMA/Weekend/story?id=3191903&page=1.

Is a sugar rush a better pick-me-up than caffeine?: C. Anderson and J. A. Horne, "A High Sugar Content, Low Caffeine Drink Does Not Alleviate Sleepiness but May Worsen It," *Human Psychopharmacology*, 21(5) (July 2006): 299–303. J. K. Wyatt et al., "Low-Dose Repeated Caffeine Administration for Circadian-Phase-Dependent Performance Degradation During Extended Wakefulness," *Sleep*, 27(3) (May 1, 2004): 374–81.

Can drinking tea reduce stress?: Statistics on workers and stress available at http://www.cdc.gov/Niosh/stresswk.html. A. Steptoe et al., "The Effects of Tea on Psychophysiological Stress Responsivity and Post-Stress Recovery: A Randomised Double-Blind Trial," *Psychopharmacology*, 190(1) (Jan. 2007): 81–89. S. Kuriyama, "The Relation Between Green Tea Consumption and Cardiovascular Disease as Evidenced by Epidemiological Studies," *Journal of Nutrition*, 138(8) (Aug. 2008): 1548S–1553S. H. Iso et al. (JACC study group), "The Relationship Between Green Tea and Total Caffeine Intake and Risk for Self-Reported Type 2 Diabetes Among Japanese Adults," *Annals of Internal Medicine*, 144(8) (Apr. 18, 2006): 554–

62. M. Inoue et al., "Green Tea Intake, MTHFR/TYMS Genotype, and Breast Cancer Risk: The Singapore Chinese Health Study," *Carcinogenesis*, 29(10) (July 31, 2008): 1967–72. I. C. Arts, "A Review of the Epidemiological Evidence on Tea, Flavonoids, and Lung Cancer," *Journal of Nutrition*, 138(8) (Aug. 2008): 1561S–66S.

Do spicy foods boost your metabolism?: "Try Hot, Spicy Foods as Diet Strategy, Researcher Says," *Canadian Press*, Nov. 14, 1997. M. S. Westerterp-Plantenga, A. Smeets, and M. P. Lejeune, "Sensory and Gastrointestinal Satiety Effects of Capsaicin on Food Intake," *International Journal of Obesity*, 29(6) (June 2005): 682–88. A. Mori et al., "Capsaicin, a Component of Red Peppers, Inhibits the Growth of Androgen-Independent, p53 Mutant Prostate Cancer Cells," *Cancer Research*, 66(6) (Mar. 15, 2006): 3222–29. See also http://www.sciencelab.com/xMSDS-Capsaicin_Natural-9923296.

Will a spicy meal before bed ruin your sleep?: S. J. Edwards et al., "Spicy Meal Disturbs Sleep: An Effect of Thermoregulation?" *International Journal of Psychophysiology*, 13(2) (Sept. 1992): 97–100. See also http://www.nlm.nih.gov/medlineplus/ency/article/003209.htm.

Is there any truth to the Freshmen 15?: D. J. Hoffman et al., "Changes in Body Weight and Fat Mass of Men and Women in the First Year of College: A Study of the 'Freshman 15,'" *Journal of the American College of Health*, 55(1) (July–Aug. 2006): 41–45. N. L. Mihalopoulos, P. Auinger, and J. D. Klein, "The Freshman 15: Is It Real?" *Journal of the American College of Health*, 56(5) (Mar.–Apr. 2008): 531–33. L. Hajhosseini et al., "Changes in Body Weight, Body Composition and Resting Metabolic Rate (RMR) in First-Year University Freshmen Students," *Journal of the American College of Nutrition*, 25(2) (Apr. 2006): 123–27. S. B. Racette et al., "Changes in Weight and Health Behaviors from Freshman Through Senior Year of College," *Journal of Nutrition Education and Behavior*, 40(1) (Jan.–Feb. 2008): 39–42.

Is there really such a thing as a runner's high?: H. Boecker et al., "The Runner's High: Opioidergic Mechanisms in the Human Brain," *Cerebral Cortex*, 18(11) (Feb. 21, 2008): 2523–31.

Does running on a treadmill burn fewer calories than running on pavement?: C. Milgrom et al., "Are Overground or Treadmill Runners More Likely to Sustain Tibial Stress Fracture?" *British Journal of Sports Medicine*, 37(2) (Apr. 2003): 160–63.

Can stretching before a workout prevent injuries?: R. D. Herbert and M. de Noronha, "Stretching to Prevent or Reduce Muscle Soreness After Exercise," *Cochrane Database of Systematic Reviews*, (4) (Oct. 17, 2007): CD004577. S. B. Thacker et al., "The Impact of Stretching on Sports Injury Risk: A Systematic Review of the Literature," *Medicine and Science in Sports and Exercise*, 36(3) (Mar. 2004): 371–78. I. Shrier, "Should People Stretch Before Exercise?" *Western Journal of Medicine*, 174(4) (Apr. 2001): 282–83.

Is it true the tongue is mapped into four areas of taste?: A. L. Huang et al., "The Cells and Logic for Mammalian Sour Taste Detection," *Nature*, 442(7105) (Aug. 24, 2006): 934–38. K. Sato, S. Endo, and H. Tomita, "Sensitivity of Three Loci on the Tongue and Soft Palate to Four Basic Tastes in Smokers and Non-smokers," *Acta Oto-Laryngologica: Supplementum*, 122(S546) (June 2002): 74–82.

4. Drink to Your Health

Introduction: Ron S. Jackson, *Wine Science: Principles, Practice, Perception* (3rd ed.) (San Diego: Academic Press, 2008). M. Laska and A. Seibt, "Olfactory Sensitivity for Aliphatic Alcohols in Squirrel Monkeys and Pigtail Macaques," *Journal of Experimental Biology*, 205(pt. 11) (June 2002): 1633–43. D. J. Chivers and P. Langer (eds.), *The Digestive System in Mammals: Food, Form, and Function* (New York: Cambridge University Press, 1994), 150–65.

Do calories from alcohol go straight to your midsection?: J. M. Dorn et al., "Alcohol Drinking Patterns Differentially Affect Central Adiposity as Measured by Abdominal Height in Women and Men," *Journal of Nutrition*, 133(8) (Aug. 2003): 2655–62.

Can alcohol warm you up in the winter?: B. J. Freund, C. O'Brien, and A. J. Young, "Alcohol Ingestion and Temperature Regulation During Cold Exposure," *Journal of Wilderness Medicine*, 5(1) (Feb. 1994): 88–98. T. Yoda et al., "Effects of Alcohol on Thermoregulation During Mild Heat Exposure in Humans," *Alcohol*, 36(3) (July 2005): 195–200. A. J. Taylor et al., "Hypothermia Deaths in Jefferson County, Alabama," *Injury Prevention*, 7(2) (June 2001): 141–45.

Can a little alcohol help you beat a cold?: S. Cohen et al., "Smoking, Alcohol Consumption, and Susceptibility to the Common Cold," *American Journal of Public Health*, 83(9) (Sept. 1993): 1277–83. B. Takkouche et al., "Intake of Wine, Beer, and Spirits and the Risk of Clinical Common Cold," *American Journal of Epidemiology*, 155(9) (May 1, 2002): 853–58.

Do you get drunk faster when you drink at higher altitudes?: E. A. Higgins, J. A. Vaughan, and G. E. Funkhouser, "Blood Alcohol Concentrations as Affected by Combinations of Alcoholic Beverage Dosages and Altitudes," *Aerospace Medicine*, 41(10) (Oct. 1970): 1129–32. E. A. Higgins et al., "The Effects of Alcohol at Three Simulated Aircraft Cabin Conditions," *Federal Aviation Administration Aviation Medicine Reports*, 68(18) (Sept. 1968): 1–14. W. E. Collins, H. W. Mertens, and E. A. Higgins, "Some Effects of Alcohol and Simulated Altitude on Complex Performance Scores and Breathalyzer Readings," *Aviation and Space Environmental Medicine*, 58(4) (Apr. 1987): 328–32. W. E. Collins and H. W. Mertens, "Age, Alcohol, and Simulated Altitude: Effects on Performance and Breathalyzer Scores," *Aviation and Space Environmental Medicine*, 59(11, pt. 1) (Nov. 1988): 1026–33.

Can some mixers make you more drunk?: K. L. Wu et al., "Artificially Sweetened versus Regular Mixers Increase Gastric Emptying and Alcohol Absorption," *American Journal of Medicine*, 119(9) (Sept. 2006): 802. C. Roberts and S. P. Robinson, "Alcohol Concentration and Carbonation of Drinks: The Effect on Blood Alcohol Levels," *Journal of Forensic Legal Medicine*, 14(7) (Oct. 2007): 398–405. Published online May 2007.

Can some types of alcohol cause worse hangovers than others?: I. Calder, "Hangovers," *British Medical Journal*, 314(7073) (Jan. 4, 1997): 2–3. G. L. Pawan, "Alcoholic Drinks and Hangover Effects," *Proceedings of the Nutrition Society*, 32(1) (May 1973): 15A.

Are there any proven hangover cures?: R. H. Ylikahri et al., "Effects of Fructose and Glucose on Ethanol-Induced Metabolic Changes and on the Intensity of Alcohol Intoxication and Hangover," *European Journal of Clinical Investigation*, 6(1) (Jan. 30, 1976): 93–102. P. Bendtsen, A. W. Jones, and A. Helander, "Urinary Excretion of Methanol and 5-hydroxytryptophol as Biochemical Markers of Recent Drinking in the Hangover State," *Alcohol*, 33(4) (July–Aug. 1998): 431–38. M. A. Khan, K. Jensen, and H. J. Krogh, "Alcohol-Induced Hangover: A Double-Blind Comparison of Pyritinol and Placebo in Preventing Hangover Symptoms," *Quarterly Journal of Studies on Alcohol*, 34(4) (Dec. 1973): 1195–201. George Ade quoted in J. G. Wiese, M. G. Shlipak, and W. S. Browner, "The Alcohol Hangover," *Annals of Internal Medicine*, 132(11) (June 6, 2000): 897–902.

Does grape juice have the same health benefits as red wine?: J. H. Stein et al., "Purple Grape Juice Improves Endothelial Function and Reduces the Susceptibility of LDL Cholesterol to Oxidation in Patients with Coronary Artery Disease," *Circulation*, 100(10) (Sept. 7, 1999): 1050–55. D. Shanmuganayagam et al., "Concord Grape Juice Attenuates Platelet Aggregation, Serum Cholesterol and Development of Atheroma in Hypercholesterolemic Rabbits," *Atherosclerosis*, 190(1) (Jan. 2007): 135–42. Published online June 14, 2006.

Can a silver spoon in a bottle of champagne keep it from going flat?: See http:// news-service.stanford.edu/pr/94/941221Arc4008.html.

Is New Year's the most dangerous time to be on the road?: C. M. Farmer and A. F. Williams, "Temporal Factors in Motor Vehicle Crash Deaths," *Injury Prevention*, 11(1) (Feb. 2005): 18–23.

5. Love Medicine

Introduction: M. Diamond et al., "Pornography, Rape and Sex Crimes in Japan," *International Journal of Law and Psychiatry*, 22 (1) (Jan. 1999): 1–22.

Can sex be substituted for a workout?: B. E. Ainsworth et al., "Compendium of Physical Activities: An Update of Activity Codes and MET Intensities," *Medicine and Science in Sports and Exercise*, 32(9 Suppl.) (Sept. 2000): S498–504. B. E. Ainsworth et al., "Compendium of Physical Activities: Classification of Energy Costs of Human Physical Activities," *Medicine and Science in Sports and Exercise*, 25(1) (Jan. 1993): 71–80.

Do short men have less luck with women?: B. Pawlowski and G. Jasienska, "Women's Preferences for Sexual Dimorphism in Height Depend on Menstrual Cycle Phase and Expected Duration of Relationship," *Biological Psychology*, 70(1) (Sept. 2005): 38–43. D. Nettle, "Height and Reproductive Success in a Cohort of British Men," *Human Nature*, 13(4) (Dec. 2002): 473–91; www.springerlink.com/content/p5ty6k1e3a69dp80.

Can being on birth control increase your chances of becoming infertile?: H. Doll, M. Vessey, and R. Painter, "Return of Fertility in Nulliparous Women After Discontinuation of the Intrauterine Device: Comparison with Women Discontinuing Other Methods of Contraception," *British Journal of Obstetrics and Gynaecology*, 108(3) (Mar. 2001): 304–14.

Will there ever be a male birth control pill?: K. Heinemann et al., "Attitudes Toward Male Fertility Control: Results of a Multinational Survey on Four Continents," *Human Reproduction*, 20(2) (Feb. 2005): 549–56.

Do women's menstrual cycles synchronize?: M. K. McClintock, "Menstrual Synchrony and Suppression," *Nature*, 229(5282) (Jan. 22, 1971): 244–45. Z. Yang and J. C. Schank, "Women Do Not Synchronize Their Menstrual Cycles," *Human Nature*, 17 (4) (Dec. 2006): 433–47. L. Weller et al., "Menstrual Synchrony in a Sample of Working Women," *Psychoneuroendocrinology*, 24(4) (May 1999): 449–59. C. Wedekind et al., "MHC-Dependent Mate Preferences in Humans," *Proceedings of the Royal Society: Biological Sciences*, 260(1359) (June 22, 1995): 245–49.

Can bicycle seats cause impotence in women?: M. K. Guess et al., "Genital Sensation and Sexual Function in Women Bicyclists and Runners: Are Your Feet Safer Than Your Seat?" *Journal of Sexual Medicine*, 3(6) (Nov. 2005): 1018–27. M. L. Chivers and J. M. Bailey, "A Sex Difference in Features That Elicit Genital Response," *Biological Psychology*, 70(2) (Oct. 2005): 115–20.

Can a woman be allergic to semen?: D. J. Resnick et al., "The Approach to Conception for Women with Seminal Plasma Protein Hypersensitivity," *American Journal of Reproductive Immunology*, 52(1) (July 2004): 42–44. S. Weidinger, "IgE-mediated Allergy Against Human Seminal Plasma," *Chemical Immunology and Allergy*, 88 (Aug. 2005): 128–38.

Can hot tubs cause infertility?: S. Shefi et al., "Wet Heat Exposure: A Potentially Reversible Cause of Low Semen Quality in Infertile Men," *Journal of the Brazilian Society of Urology*, 33(1) (Jan.–Feb. 2007): 50–56; discussion 56–57. D. K. Li et al., "Hot Tub Use During Pregnancy and the Risk of Miscarriage," *American Journal of Epidemiology*, 158(10) (Nov. 15, 2003): 931–37.

Do Kegel exercises work?: S. Hagen et al., "Conservative Management of Pelvic Organ Prolapse in Women," *Cochrane Database of Systematic Reviews*, (4) (Oct. 18, 2006): CD003882. J. Belo et al., "Pelvic Floor Muscle Training with Plevnik's Cones in Women with Urinary Incontinence," *Acta Médica Portuguesa*, 18(2) (Mar.–Apr. 2005): 117–22. N. Baum and B. Spieler, "Medical Management of Premature Ejaculation," *Medical Aspects of Human Sexuality*, 29 (May 2001): 15–25.

Are two condoms better protection than one?: Planned Parenthood statistics at www.plannedparenthood.org/health-topics/birth-control/condom -10187.htm#effective. National Institutes of Health report on STD/ condom risk at http://www3.niaid.nih.gov/about/organization/dmid/ PDF/condomReport.pdf. R. Crosby et al., "Condom Misuse Among Adjudicated Girls: Associations with Laboratory-Confirmed Chlamydia and Gonorrhea," *Journal of Pediatric and Adolescent Gynecology*, 20(6) (Dec. 2007): 339–43. R. J. Wolitski et al., "Awareness and Use of Untested Barrier Methods by HIV-Seropositive Gay and Bisexual Men," *AIDS Education and Prevention*, 13(4) (Aug. 2001): 291–301.

Can a woman get pregnant during her period?: A. J. Wilcox, D. Dunson, and D. D. Baird, "The Timing of the 'Fertile Window' in the Menstrual Cycle: Day Specific Estimates from a Prospective Study," *British Medical Journal*, 321(7271) (Nov. 18, 2000): 1259–62.

Does circumcision reduce sexual pleasure?: K. S. Fink et al., "Adult Circumcision Outcomes Study: Effect on Erectile Function, Penile Sensitivity, Sexual Activity and Satisfaction," *Journal of Urology*, 167(5) (May 2002): 2113–16. S. Masood et al., "Penile Sensitivity and Sexual Satisfaction After Circumcision: Are We Informing Men Correctly?" *Urologia Internationalis*, 75(1) (July 2005): 62–66. J. N. Krieger et al., "Adult Male Circumcision: Effects on Sexual Function and Sexual Satisfaction in Kisumu, Kenya," *Journal of Sexual Medicine*, 5(11) (Aug. 28, 2008): 2610–22(13). American Academy of Family Physicians report at www.aafp.org/online/en/home/clinical/clinicalrecs/circumcision.html.

6. Sperm Meets Egg

Does mother's heartburn mean a hairy newborn?: K. A. Costigan, H. L. Sipsma, and J. A. DiPietro, "Pregnancy Folklore Revisited: The Case of Heartburn and Hair," *Birth*, 33(4) (Dec. 2006): 311–14.

Can sexual position during conception determine a baby's sex?: R. H. Gray, "Natural Family Planning and Sex Selection: Fact or Fiction?" *American Journal of Obstetrics and Gynecology*, 165(6 pt. 2) (Dec. 1991): 1982–84. A. J. Wilcox, C. R. Weinberg, and D. D. Baird, "Timing of Sexual Intercourse in Relation to Ovulation: Effects on the Probability of Conception, Survival of the Pregnancy, and Sex of the Baby," *New England Journal of Medicine*, 333(23) (Dec. 7, 1995): 1517–21.

Can you predict the sex of a baby by the way the mother is carrying?: D. F. Perry, J. DiPietro, and K. Costigan, "Are Women Carrying 'Basketballs' Really Having Boys? Testing Pregnancy Folklore," *Birth*, 26(3) (Sept. 1999): 172–77.

Is morning sickness a sign of a healthy pregnancy? Does it mean a greater likelihood of having a girl?: N. Maconochie et al., "Risk Factors for First Trimester Miscarriage—Results from a UK-Population-Based Case-

Control Study," *British Journal of Obstetrics and Gynaecology*, 114(2) (Feb. 2007): 170–86. M. M. Weigel et al., "Is the Nausea and Vomiting of Early Pregnancy Really Feto-Protective?" *Journal of Perinatal Medicine*, 34(2) (Apr. 2006): 115–22. S. M. Flaxman and P. W. Sherman, "Morning Sickness: A Mechanism for Protecting Mother and Embryo," *Quarterly Review of Biology*, 75(2) (June 2000): 113–48. M. A. Schiff, S. D. Reed, and J. R. Daling, "The Sex Ratio of Pregnancies Complicated by Hospitalisation for Hyperemesis Gravidarum," *British Journal of Obstetrics and Gynaecology*, 111(1) (Jan. 2004): 27–30. J. Askling et al., "Sickness in Pregnancy and Sex of Child," *Lancet*, 354(9195) (Dec. 11, 1999): 2053. M. del Mar Melero-Montes and H. Jick, "Hyperemesis Gravidarum and the Sex of the Offspring," *Epidemiology*, 12(1) (Jan. 2001): 123–24. P. C. Tan et al., "The Fetal Sex Ratio and Metabolic, Biochemical, Haematological and Clinical Indicators of Severity of Hyperemesis Gravidarum," *British Journal of Obstetrics and Gynaecology*, 113(6) (June 2006): 733–37.

Can fetal heart rate predict the sex of the baby?: O. Oguch and P. Steer, "Gender Does Not Affect Fetal Heart Rate Variation," *British Journal of Obstetrics and Gynaecology*, 105(12) (Dec. 1998): 1312–14.

Do identical twins have identical DNA?: C. E. Bruder et al., "Phenotypically Concordant and Discordant Monozygotic Twins Display Different DNA Copy-Number-Variation Profiles," *American Journal of Human Genetics*, 82(3) (Mar. 2008): 763–71.

Does a new mother really lose a tooth and gain a child?: See www.nyu.edu/ public.affairs/releases/detail/224. M. L. Gaffield et al., "Oral Health During Pregnancy: An Analysis of Information Collected by the Pregnancy Risk Assessment Monitoring System," *Journal of the American Dental Association*, 132(7) (July 2001): 1009–16.

Is a baby's fever just a sign of teething?: M. L. Macknin et al., "Symptoms Associated with Infant Teething: A Prospective Study," *Pediatrics*, 105(4 pt. 1) (Apr. 2000): 747–52.

Will rubbing alcohol help cool a baby's fever?: L. C. Smitherman, J. Janisse, and A. Mathur, "The Use of Folk Remedies Among Children in an Urban Black Community: Remedies for Fever, Colic, and Teething," *Pediatrics*, 115(3) (Mar. 2005): e297–304. M. Arditi and M. S. Killner, "Coma Following Use of Rubbing Alcohol for Fever Control," *American Journal of Diseases of Children*, 141(3) (Mar. 1987): 237–78.

Do babies blink less than adults?: A. J. Zametkin et al., "Annals of Neurology Study: Ontogeny of Spontaneous Blinking and of Habituation of the Blink Reflex," *Annals of Neurology*, 5(5) (May 1979): 453–57.

7. Attack of the Body Invaders

Should you feed a cold and starve a fever?: G. R. van den Brink et al., "Feed a Cold, Starve a Fever?" *Clinical and Diagnostic Laboratory Immunology*, 9(1) (Jan. 2002): 182–83.

Can a cup of tea clear up your chest?: A. Sanu and R. Eccles, "The Effects of a Hot Drink on Nasal Airflow and Symptoms of Common Cold and Flu," *Rhinology*, 46(4) (Dec. 2008): 271–75. E. Ernst et al., "Regular Sauna Bathing and the Incidence of Common Colds," *Annals of Medicine*, 22(4) (1990): 225–27.

Can taking zinc help you beat a cold?: R. B. Turner and W. E. Cetnarowski, "Effect of Treatment with Zinc Gluconate or Zinc Acetate on Experimental and Natural Colds," *Clinical and Infectious Diseases*, 31(5) (Nov. 2000): 1202–8. T. J. Caruso, C. G. Prober, and J. M. Gwaltney Jr., "Treatment of Naturally Acquired Common Colds with Zinc: A Structured Review," *Clinical and Infectious Diseases*, 45(5) (Sept. 1, 2007): 569–74.

Is it a cold? Is it an allergy? How can you tell the difference?: S. Croner, Genetics and Allergies Study: Prediction and Detection of Allergy Development: Influence of Genetic and Environmental Factors, *Journal of Pediatrics*, 121 (5 pt. 2) (Nov. 1992): S58–63.

Is drinking hot water from the tap bad for you?: R. P. Maas, S. C. Patch, and A. F. Parker, "An Assessment of Lead Exposure Potential from Residential Cutoff Valves," *Journal of Environmental Health*, 65(1) (July–Aug. 2002): 9–14, 28.

Should you always cool hot leftovers at room temperature?: CDC, *Mortality and Morbidity Weekly Report*, 43(8) (Mar. 4, 1994): 137–38, 143–44.

Are public restrooms as filthy as everyone thinks they are?: Reuters, "Flushing Out the Truth About Public Restrooms," May 22, 2008. K. A. Reynolds et al., "Occurrence of Bacteria and Biochemical Markers on Public Surfaces," *International Journal of Environmental Health Research*, 15(3) (June 2005): 225–34.

Can you disinfect a kitchen sponge by microwaving it?: See http://thurston .wsu.edu/Food%20Safety/Kitchen%20Clean%20Up/sponges%20 and%20wiping%20cloths%204-22-98.htm. D. K. Park, G. Bitton, and R. Melker, "Microbial Inactivation by Microwave Radiation in the Home Environment," *Journal of Environmental Health*, 69(5) (Dec. 2006): 17–24; quiz 39–40. B. G. Border and L. Rice-Spearman, "Microwaves in the Laboratory: Effective Decontamination," *Clinical Laboratory Science*, 12(3) (May–June 1999): 156–60.

Does double-dipping spread germs?: See www.clemson.edu/foodscience/PDF %20Downloads/Double-Dipping%20Does%20Transfer%20Bacteria.pdf.

Is there any truth to the five-second rule?: P. Dawson et al., "Residence Time and Food Contact Time Effects on Transfer of *Salmonella typhimurium* from Tile, Wood and Carpet: Testing the Five-Second Rule," *Journal of Applied Microbiology*, 102(4) (Apr. 2007): 945–53.

8. Hi, Technology

Can you stand too close to your microwave oven?: Microwave Oven Radiation, Center for Devices and Radiological Health Consumer Information, U.S. Food and Drug Administration, http://www.fda.gov/cdrh/ consumer/microwave.html.

Is it true that you should never use a cell phone on an airplane?: Bill Strauss et al., "Unsafe at Any Airspeed?" *IEEE Spectrum*, 43(3) (Mar. 2006): 44–49, www .spectrum.ieee.org/print/3069.

What about cell phones in hospitals?: Associated Press, "Man Arrested After Refusing to Stop Using Cell Phone in Hospital," Nov. 26, 1998. J. L. Tri et al., "Use of Cellular Telephones in the Hospital Environment," *Mayo Clinic Proceedings*, 82(3) (Mar. 2007): 282–85. E. J. van Lieshout et al., "Interference by New-Generation Mobile Phones on Critical Care Medical Equipment," *Critical Care*, 11(5) (Sept. 2007): R98.

Is hospital care worse on weekends?: W. J. Kostis et al., Myocardial Infarction Data Acquisition System (MIDAS 10) Study Group, "Weekend versus Weekday Admission and Mortality from Myocardial Infarction," *New England Journal of Medicine*, 356(11) (Mar. 15, 2007): 1099–109. M. M. Zare et al., "Mortality After Nonemergent Major Surgery Performed on Friday versus Monday through Wednesday," *Annals of Surgery*, 246(5) (Nov. 2007): 866–74.

Do computer keyboards cause carpal tunnel syndrome?: National Institutes of Health, www.ninds.nih.gov/disorders/carpal_tunnel/detail_carpal _tunnel.htm. J. C. Stevens et al., "The Frequency of Carpal Tunnel

Syndrome in Computer Users at a Medical Facility," *Neurology*, 56 (June 2001): 1568–70.

Does cold water boil more quickly than hot water?: Aristotle, *Meteorologica* (Cambridge, Mass.: Harvard University Press, 1962), book 1, 85–87. M. Jeng, "The Mpemba Effect: When Can Hot Water Freeze Faster Than Cold?" *American Journal of Physics*, 74(6) (June 2006): 514. See http://scitation.aip.org/ajp.arxiv.org/abs/physics/0604224v1.

What's the safest seat in a car?: J. Mayrose, "The Effect of Unrestrained Rear-Seat Passengers on Driver Mortality," *Journal of Trauma*, 61(5) (Nov. 2006): 1249–54.

Do some people dream in black and white?: M. Schredl et al., "Typical Dreams: Stability and Gender Differences," *Journal of Psychology*, 138(6) (Nov. 2004): 485–94. E. Murzyn, "Do We Only Dream in Colour? A Comparison of Reported Dream Colour in Younger and Older Adults with Different Experiences of Black and White Media," *Consciousness and Cognition*, 17(4) (Dec. 2008): 1228–37. E. Schwitzgebel, "Do People Still Report Dreaming in Black and White? An Attempt to Replicate a Questionnaire from 1942," *Perceptual and Motor Skills*, 96(1) (Feb. 2003): 25–29. C. Hurovitz et al., "The Dreams of Blind Men and Women: A Replication and Extension of Previous Findings," *Dreaming*, 9(2–3) (June 1999): 183–93.

9. Weathering the Elements

Does darker skin better protect you against skin cancer?: J. N. Cormier et al., "Ethnic Differences Among Patients with Cutaneous Melanoma," *Archives of Internal Medicine*, 166(17) (Sept. 25, 2006): 1907–14. S. Hu et al., "Comparison of Stage at Diagnosis of Melanoma Among Hispanic, Black, and White Patients in Miami–Dade County, Florida," *Archives of Dermatology*, 42(6) (June 2006): 704–8. American Academy of Dermatology, 2005 Skin Cancer Survey Fact Sheet, www.aad.org.

Are high SPF ratings really better?: A. Faurschou and H. C. Wulf, "The Relation Between Sun Protection Factor and Amount of Sunscreen Applied in Vivo," *British Journal of Dermatology*, 156(4) (Apr. 2007): 716–19.

Can the chlorine in pools cause hair loss?: H. Nanko et al., "Hair-Discoloration of Japanese Elite Swimmers," *Journal of Dermatology*, 27(10) (Oct. 2000): 625–34. J. L. Escartin et al., "A Study of Dental Staining Among Competitive Swimmers," *Community Dentistry and Oral Epidemiology*, 28(1) (Feb. 2000): 10–17.

Can eating garlic ward off mosquitoes? What about vitamin B?: T. V. Rajan et al., "A Double-Blinded, Placebo-Controlled Trial of Garlic as a Mosquito Repellant: A Preliminary Study," *Medical and Veterinary Entomology*, 19(1) (Mar. 2005): 84–89. A. R. Ives and S. M. Paskewitz, "Testing Vitamin B as a Home Remedy Against Mosquitoes," *Journal of the American Mosquito Control Association*, 21(2) (June 2005): 213–17. M. F. Silva et al., "Experimental Evaluation in Mice of Vitamin B Complex Repellent Activity Against *Culex quinquefasciatus*," *Revista do Hospital das Clínicas, Faculdade de Medicina da Universidade de São Paulo*, 50(1) (Jan.–Feb. 1995): 55–57; in Portuguese. O. Shirai, "Alcohol Ingestion Stimulates Mosquito Attraction," *Journal of the American Mosquito Control Association*, 18(2) (June 2002): 91–96.

Does a person struck by lightning retain an electrical charge?: Statistics and figures provided by the National Oceanic and Atmospheric Administration and the Tropical Rainfall Measurement Mission Satellite.

Can thunderstorms cause asthma attacks?: A. Grundstein, "Thunderstorm Associated Asthma in Atlanta, Georgia," *Thorax*, 63(7) (July 2008): 659–60.

Do changes in the weather cause heart attacks?: C. L. Chang, "Lower Ambient Temperature Was Associated with an Increased Risk of Hospitalization for Stroke and Acute Myocardial Infarction in Young Women," *Journal of Clinical Epidemiology*, 57(7) (July 2004): 749–57. European Society of Cardiology Congress, Munich, Germany, Aug. 28–Sept. 1, 2004. T. S. Field and M. D. Hill, "Weather, Chinook, and Stroke Occurrence," *Stroke*, 33(7) (July 2002): 1751–57.

Can mistletoe be deadly? What about poinsettias?: H. A. Spiller et al., "Retrospective Study of Mistletoe Ingestion," *Journal of Toxicology: Clinical Toxicology*, 34(4) (1996): 405–8. E. P. Krenzelok, T. D. Jacobsen, and J. M. Aronis, "Poinsettia Exposures Have Good Outcomes . . . Just as We Thought," *American Journal of Emergency Medicine*, 14(7) (Nov. 1996): 671–74.

10. World Health

Can animals tell when a natural disaster is about to strike? Do they have a sixth sense?: Study of Yala National Park at www.iisc.ernet.in/currsci/jun102006/1531.pdf. Stanford report article at http://news-service.stanford.edu/news/2005/june1/elephant-052505.html.

Does early to bed, early to rise, make a man healthy, wealthy, and wise?: Dame

Berners quoted in Wolfgang Mieder, "De Proverbio: An Electronic Journal of International Proverb Studies," www.deproverbio.com/DPjournal/DP,1,1,95/FRANKLIN.html. C. Gale and C. Martyn, "Larks and Owls and Health, Wealth, and Wisdom," *British Medical Journal*, 317(7174) (Dec. 19–26, 1998): 1675–77. K. J. Mukamal, G. A. Wellenius, and M. A. Mittleman, "Early to Bed and Early to Rise: Does It Matter?" *Canadian Medical Association Journal*, 175(12) (Dec. 5, 2006): 1560–62.

Can honey soothe a cough and other respiratory ailments?: www.sciencedaily .com/releases/2008/09/080923091335.htm. I. M. Paul et al., "Effect of Honey, Dextromethorphan, and No Treatment on Nocturnal Cough and Sleep Quality for Coughing Children and Their Parents," *Archives of Pediatric and Adolescent Medicine*, 161(12) (Dec. 2007): 1140–46.

Can pomegranates increase virility?: P. Langley, "Why a Pomegranate?" *British Medical Journal*, 321(7269) (Nov. 4, 2000): 1153–54. G. Türk et al., "Effects of Pomegranate Juice Consumption on Sperm Quality, Spermatogenic Cell Density, Antioxidant Activity and Testosterone Level in Male Rats," *Clinical Nutrition*, 27(2) (Apr. 2008): 289–96. Published online Jan. 28, 2008.

Are those açai berry drinks all they're cracked up to be?: E. M. Kuskoski et al., "Wild Fruits and Pulps of Frozen Fruits: Antioxidant Activity, Polyphenols and Anthocyanins," *Ciência Rural*, 36(4) (July–Aug. 2006): 1283–87. A. G. Schauss et al., "Açai Berries as COX Inhibitor: Antioxidant Capacity and Other Bioactivities of the Freeze-Dried Amazonian Palm Berry, *Euterpe oleraceae mart.* (Açai)," *Journal of Agricultural and Food Chemistry*, 54(22) (Nov. 1, 2006): 8604–10. D. Del Pozo-Insfran, S. S. Percival, and S. T. Talcott, "Açai (*Euterpe oleracea mart.*) Polyphenolics in Their Glycoside and Aglycone Forms Induce Apoptosis of HL-60 Leukemia Cells," *Journal of Agricultural and Food Chemistry*, 54(4) (Feb. 22, 2006): 1222–29.

Is Guinness good for your health?: K. Berger et al., "Light-to-Moderate Alcohol Consumption and Risk of Stroke Among U.S. Male Physicians," *New England Journal of Medicine*, 341(21) (Nov. 18, 1999): 1557–64. L. B. Mann and J. D. Folts, "Effects of Ethanol and Other Constituents of Alcoholic Beverages on Coronary Heart Disease: A Review," *Pathophysiology*, 10(2) (Apr. 2004): 105–12.

Can eating licorice raise your blood pressure?: H. A. Sigurjónsdóttir et al., "Liquorice-Induced Rise in Blood Pressure: A Linear Dose-Response Relationship," *Journal of Human Hypertension*, 15(8) (Aug. 2001): 549–52.

Woman eats too much licorice reference: BBC News online, "Woman overdoses on licorice," May 21, 2004.

Why was there an explosion in male babies in postwar Europe?: C. Gellatly, "Trends in Population Sex Ratios May Be Explained by Changes in the Frequencies of Polymorphic Alleles of a Sex Ratio Gene," *Evolutionary Biology*, Dec. 2008; DOI: 10.1007/s11692-008-9046-3, http://www.springerlink.com/content/d87k212rx7l7211g/.

Can hot peppers cure an ulcer?: K. G. Yeoh et al., "Chile Protects Against Aspirin-Induced Gastroduodenal Mucosal Injury in Humans," *Digestive Diseases and Sciences*, 40(3) (Mar. 1995): 580–83. M. N. Satyanarayana, "Capsaicin and Gastric Ulcers," *Critical Reviews in Food Science and Nutrition*, 46(4) (June 2006): 275–328. T. P. Ng et al., "Curry Consumption and Cognitive Function in the Elderly," *American Journal of Epidemiology*, 164(9) (Nov. 1, 2006): 898–906.

Epilogue

Exercizing the brain: K. Ball et al., "Effects of Cognitive Training Interventions with Older Adults: A Randomized Controlled Trial," *Journal of the American Medical Association*, 288(18) (Nov. 13, 2002): 2271–81.

ACKNOWLEDGMENTS

Yet again, I must begin by thanking groups of people without whom the "Really?" column would not exist: the scientists who take on old wives' tales and other puzzles of modern health and healthy living and the many fans of the *New York Times* column. Without your answers and your questions, the "Really?" bit would be far less entertaining and thought-provoking.

As I mentioned in my thanks in *Never Shower in a Thunderstorm*, the column itself would not have been possible without the inspiration and support of my editor at Science Times, Erica Goode. I am grateful to Alex Ward, the director of book development at the *Times*, and to Robin Dennis, my editor at Times Books, both of whom helped to make this book (as well as *Never Shower in a Thunderstorm*) better. At Henry Holt, Chris O'Connell, Meryl Levavi, Emi Ikkanda, and Dana Trombley have made this book as much fun as the last one. Thanks as well to my agent, Christy Fletcher, and to Leif Parsons, whose excellent illustrations bring to life the cover and chapters of this book.

Once again, my friends and loved ones served as sounding boards, punch line generators, and writing relief, and I'd like to single out Garren, Dave, Steve, and Alexandra for being there for book number two. My mom, Karen, and the rest of my family always give me their unconditional support and encouragement. Thank you.

Finally, thank you to my editor at the *New York Times*, David Corcoran, and to everyone else at the paper whose brilliance and dedication to journalism make working at the *Times* a dream come true.

INDEX

ABOUT THE AUTHOR

ANAHAD O'CONNOR is a reporter for the *New York Times* covering breaking national news and contributes the weekly column "Really?"—named for his favorite word in journalism—to the paper's Science Times section. The author of *Never Shower in a Thunderstorm*, he lives in New York City.